The Psychological Experience of Surgery

WILEY SERIES IN GENERAL AND CLINICAL PSYCHIATRY

The Broad Scope of Ego Function Assessment
Edited by Leopold Bellak and Lisa A. Goldsmith

The Psychological Experience of Surgery
Edited by Richard S. Blacher

THE PSYCHOLOGICAL
EXPERIENCE OF SURGERY

Edited by

Richard S. Blacher, M.D.

A Wiley-Interscience Publication

JOHN WILEY & SONS

New York • Chichester • Brisbane • Toronto • Singapore

Copyright © 1987 by John Wiley & Sons, Inc.

All rights reserved. Published simultaneously in Canada.

Reproduction or translation of any part of this work
beyond that permitted by Section 107 or 108 of the
1976 United States Copyright Act without the permission
of the copyright owner is unlawful. Requests for
permission or further information should be addressed to
the Permissions Department, John Wiley & Sons, Inc.

Library of Congress Cataloging in Publication Data:

The psychological experience of surgery.

(Wiley series in general and clinical psychiatry)
"A Wiley-Interscience publication."
Includes indexes.
1. Surgery—Psychological aspects. I. Blacher,
Richard S. II. Series. [DNLM: 1. Surgery, Operative—
psychology. WO 500 P9742]

RD31.7.P78 1986   617   86-11124
ISBN   0-471-81831-3

Printed in the United States of America

10 9 8 7 6 5 4 3 2 1

Contributors

SAMUEL H. BASCH, M.D.
Clinical Associate Professor of
  Psychiatry
Mount Sinai School of Medicine
New York, New York

NORMAN R. BERNSTEIN, M.D.
Professor of Psychiatry
University of Illinois
Chicago, Illinois

RICHARD S. BLACHER, M.D.
Professor of Psychiatry
Lecturer in Surgery
Tufts University School of Medicine
Boston, Massachusetts

PIETRO CASTELNUOVO-TEDESCO,
  M.D.
Blakemore Professor of Psychiatry
Vanderbilt University School
  of Medicine
Nashville, Tennessee

JOSEPH JAFFE, M.D.
Professor of Clinical Psychiatry
  (in Neurological Surgery)
College of Physicians & Surgeons of
  Columbia University
New York, New York

LOUIS LINN, M.D.
Clinical Professor Emeritus of
  Psychiatry
Mount Sinai School of Medicine
Consultant Psychiatrist
Mount Sinai Hospital
New York, New York

BERNARD C. MEYER, M.D.
Professor of Clinical Psychiatry
  Emeritus
Mount Sinai School of Medicine
Attending Psychiatrist
Mount Sinai Hospital
New York, New York

MALKAH T. NOTMAN, M.D.
Professor of Psychiatry
Tufts University School of Medicine
Boston, Massachusetts

JUDITH ELLEN ROBINSON, M.D.
Assistant Professor of Psychiatry
Tufts University School of Medicine
Director of Inpatient Child
  Psychiatry Service
New England Medical Center
Boston, Massachusetts

MARY JANE SCHIRGER-KREBS, R.N.
Researcher in Psychiatry
Cornell University Medical Center
New York Hospital
New York, New York

LAURIE A. STEVENS, M.D.
Assistant Clinical Professor of
  Psychiatry
College of Physicians and
  Surgeons
Attending Psychiatrist
Department of Consultation/
  Liaison Psychiatry
Columbia Presbyterian Medical
  Center
New York, New York

PETER G. WILSON, M.D.
Associate Professor of Psychiatry
Cornell University Medical
  Center
Attending Psychiatrist
New York Hospital
New York, New York

For Amy, David, Lisa, and Rick,
and of course for Maggie

Foreword

As is true for any good physician, the surgeon is full of curiosity about his patients. However, a number of elements join to derail this curiosity. On the surgeon's side, the pressures of taking scalpel to body and exploring and even seeming to mutilate the very person he is trying to help may make him hesitate to know the patient too intimately. From the patient's point of view, his need to trust the surgeon and perhaps idealize him as a miracle worker makes it almost impossible to question him or raise issues which the patient feels the surgeon will dislike or ridicule.

The authors of this book, in their role as liaison psychiatrists, have the skills and capacity to talk with patients concerning their fears — rational and irrational — about surgery. The exchange is one rarely open to the surgeon. Thus, these pages answer questions that will allow us to understand what our patients *really* go through — not what they so often blandly present to us, their attending physicians. Some of the material presented in this volume will surprise the surgical reader; some chapters will make surgeons aware that their previous sense of what the patient is going through was too vague. As in a drawing, the shading not only provides detail but may make the outline come alive, and these psychological insights will help us understand why we "knew" but didn't quite understand some patient reactions. Such insights will not only satisfy our curiosity but may be the basis for a useful understanding of our patient's plight.

RICHARD J. CLEVELAND, M.D.

Professor and Chairman
Department of Surgery
Tufts University School of Medicine

Preface

Surgery is one of life's most frightening experiences, and even operations considered minor by the physician may evoke significant psychic reactions. While surgery is a major event in a person's life, often the most important event, it may be just an everyday occasion for the physician, who therefore may have difficulty understanding why the surgical experience has such a profound effect on the patient.

It is no wonder that patients entering the operating room for surgery have difficulty maintaining psychic equilibrium. They are confronted—sometimes suddenly, sometimes electively—with the dangers of anesthesia and surgery, and then with the vicissitudes of the postoperative period. The fantasies evoked in anticipation are usually worse than reality. Anesthesia may be equated with death; surgery may stir up anxieties concerning castration, mutilation, and bizarre anatomical procedures. And overriding all surgery is the sense that an operation is an exploration that might lead to the discovery of unwanted and terrifying diseases. In many ways the fantasies stirred up by the experience may have a greater impact on patients than the actual medical situation.

Although psychiatric complications of surgery were described by Baron Dupuytren as long ago as 1834, the modern interest in how patients deal with surgery dates to Menninger's discussion of polysurgical addiction (1934). He described patients who, while not obviously abnormal, seemed to be driven to risk death by seeking multiple operations. Later articles by Ebaugh (1937) and Cobb and McDermott (1938) and classical articles by Deutsch (1942) and Meyer (1958) looked at the surgical patient both from the descriptive and psychodynamic point of view. Books by Janis (1958) and Titchener and Levine (1960) and also volumes edited by Howells (1976) and Guerra and Andrete (1980) have all discussed the underlying struggles of the patient. In recent years the horizons of surgery have expanded. New procedures confront the patient with new emotional challenges. This book will look at some of the psychological problems the patient now faces, and seeks to expand on and extend the observations of the past.

The writers share an interest in the *meaning* of the experience to the patient. A general principle we subscribe to would be that in psychology, as in all of medicine, there is always a cause for any result. The cause may be organic or psychological (or in most cases both together), and the medical attendant must try to identify significant factors. While we would not minimize the importance of brain function, we feel that psychological reactions cannot be understood as a random series of neuronal discharges. Depression and anxiety on the surgical floor do not "just happen."

The biopsychosocial approach, which Engel (1977) has emphasized, is an attempt to overcome the either-or attitude which has plagued the psychological care of patients over the years. The selective emphasis on psyche *or* soma has been most unfortunate, since it is clear that both aspects are important in describing human behavior. The recent neuropsychopharmacological revolution has made enormous strides in helping to elucidate the biological bases of human behavior. While it is difficult to imagine mental functioning without a brain, it seems clear that the biological, chemical, and electrical understanding of brain function that we possess at this point in our scientific history is not enough to help us understand much of human behavior.

The neuropsychopharmacological revolution has not served the surgical patient well. In recent years more workers in liaison psychiatry have focused on the treatment of patients with drugs, since the new medications have allowed for the relief of anxiety and major psychic upheavals in a way not previously possible. However, this has often been carried out at the expense of understanding what the patient is going through. Thus, the symptom rather than the underlying cause may be treated. Many psychiatrists, especially newly trained ones, now tend to treat the patient in a purely pharmacological way, undermining rather than enhancing the biopsychosocial approach. The patient is treated as if he were not an individual with an active intrapsychic life, but rather as a "case." In addition, there is a current tendency for those interested in the psychodynamic point of view to move away from medical matters, and we join Hawkins (1982) in decrying this trend. If the dynamic psychiatrist assumes a diminished role in the education of junior colleagues, then there may be an even greater emphasis on brain function in the future, and a lessened interest in the patient as a person. The writers of this volume would like to help redress this difficulty.

We attempt to look at how patients themselves experience the surgery. This is the unifying thread in all of the chapters. Although the styles of the papers may be different, the interest in the psychosocial meaning to patients unites them. I recognize that there are some omissions. Areas of surgery such as heart and liver transplantation have been omitted although some of the issues of transplantation have been discussed.

Concerning the style, a decision was made to use *he* rather than the more clumsy he/she in referring to patients and medical colleagues, and we hope that the reader will understand that this is not a sexist position.

I have many people to acknowledge in the putting together of this book. Maurice Green was the prime stimulus for its getting started and has served in the background as a gentle goad. Herb Reich has also pushed the project forward in great measure. I would like to thank my teachers of the past (two of whom have contributed chapters) and my students of the past and present for stimulating me to think. It goes without saying that some of our greatest teachers have been the patients who, in exchange for our trying to help them, have taught us so much when we were willing to listen. I would like to thank the surgeons with whom I have worked, for sharing their patients with me. Doctors Richard J. Cleveland, Allan Callow, Ralph Deterling, Randolph Reinhold, Sang Cho, Harold Rheinlander, Benedict Daly, Douglas Payne, and the other members of the cardiothoracic surgery team at Tufts New England Medical Center all understand that patients are people and need more than good operative technique and metabolic balance when they undergo surgery. My colleagues on the Consultation/Liaison Service of the New England Medical Center have been a much appreciated source of support and stimulation over the years. Finally, I would especially like to thank Lisa Lamorticelli, who has done a great deal more than merely type the manuscript. She has edited, suggested, and generally been a presence in the formation of this book.

RICHARD S. BLACHER, M.D.

Boston, Massachusetts
December 1986

REFERENCES

Cobb, S., & McDermott, N. T. (1938, May). Postoperative psychosis. *Medical Clinics of North America,* 569–576.

Deutsch, H. (1942). Some psychoanalytic observations in surgery. *Psychosomatic Medicine, 4;* 105.

Dupuytren, Baron Guillaume. (1834). On nervous delerium. *Lancet,* 919–923.

Ebaugh, F. G. (1937). Psychiatric complications in surgery. *Bulletin of the American College of Surgery, 22;* 153.

Engel, G. L. (1977). The need for a new medical model. *Science, 196;* 129.

Guerra, F., & Aldrete, J. A. (Eds.) (1980). *Emotional and psychological responses to anesthesia and surgery.* New York: Grune & Stratton.

Hawkins, D. R. (1982). The role of psychoanalysis in consultation-liaison psychiatry. *Psychosomatics, 23;* 1113.

Howells, J. G. (Ed.) (1976). *Modern perspectives in the psychiatric aspects of surgery.* New York: Brunner/Mazel.

Janis, I. L. (1958). *Psychological stress Psychoanalytic and behavioral studies of surgical patients.* New York: Wiley.

Menninger, K. (1934). Polysurgery and polysurgical addiction. *Psychoanalytic Quarterly, 3;* 173.

Meyer, B. C. (1958). Some psychiatric aspects of surgical practice. *Psychosomatic Medicine, 20;* 203.

Titchener, J. L., & Levine, M. (1960). *Surgery as a human experience.* New York: Oxford University Press.

Contents

The Psychological
Experience of Surgery

CHAPTER ONE

General Surgery and Anesthesia: The Emotional Experience

RICHARD S. BLACHER, M.D.

From the point of view of the patient, surgery is an extraordinary enterprise. While to the surgeon an operation is an everyday occurrence, for the patient undergoing surgery it may be the most profound incident in his life. It is not strange that patients have emotional reactions, sometimes serious ones, to their surgical experience; what is striking is that dramatic reactions are relatively infrequent. In this chapter I will propose the hypothesis that important psychological reactions are more common than the physician realizes, and that an appreciation of these responses may spell the difference between recovery and chronic illness, suffering and relative ease, and even on occasion between life and death. An understanding about how patients feel about these matters, and how they commonly react, is thus more than a matter of being kind and understanding.

It is evident that physicians and patients look upon illness, and especially

1

upon surgery, in different ways. This seems to be based on a number of different factors.

GENERAL CONSIDERATIONS

As part of their training, physicians have acquired a corpus of information that average patients cannot have at their disposal. For example, I have seen numbers of patients who have avoided herniorrhaphy surgery because of a fear that during such a procedure the testes are in danger, since examination for a hernia involves palpation in the scrotum. While the surgeon knows that this is not an issue he may not even think that the patient would have such a concern. Following herniorraphy, it is not unusual for patients to inquire "What did they find?" clearly indicating a concern about malignancy. This occurs not only in the uneducated but in the sophisticated and knowledgeable patient as well. Another dissonance in knowledge occurs when a surgeon comments on the operative area while the patient looks at his cut skin bristling with clips or black thread and strange looking drains. He has an eerie feeling of unreality when he tries to reconcile his perception with the surgeon's comment that the incision looks "beautiful." He has no way of knowing that the surgeon's experience provides different information from his and thus the wound which looks ghastly to him may indeed look fine from a technical point of view.

Perhaps the most common area of difficulty in the sharing of knowledge between patient and surgeon occurs in the language we employ. Not only does the jargon of the physician at times confuse the patient, but the medical terms used may have different meanings in technical usage and in the vernacular. The cardiologist's concern with "heart block" may be interpreted by the patient in a variety of frightening ways. To the physician, the term describes an electrocardiographic finding; for most patients the term evokes an image of obstruction of the flow of blood through the heart. To the patient, "heart failure" implies a terminal cardiac state, and "a hole in the heart" conjures up visions of blood flowing through the myocardial wall into the body cavities. For most patients, a "plastic valve" evokes the thought of cheap breakable toys.

A middle-aged accountant was seen in the intensive care unit (ICU) following intestinal surgery. She asked her physician what she might expect in the near future in terms of care. The surgeon calmly told her that she should expect to stay in the ICU a few days and then if things went well, as expected, she would be "back on the floor" after that time. With dilated pupils the patient gasped "on the floor?!," indicating she did not understand that what the surgeon meant by "floor" was the regular part of the hospital.

The physician thinks of bodily functions and illness in anatomic, physio-logic, and pathologic terms. The patient looks on illness as a quasi-magical event. Illness is also experienced as a moral issue, Witness the 90-year-old man who proudly states that he has never been ill a day in his life. This is not an expression of appreciation for his good luck in having acquired such genes, but rather a statement as to his moral superiority. In a like manner, it is not unusual for patients to respond to being told of a serious diagnosis with the statement "Why me?!," indicating that since they had led good and decent lives it was not fair to be punished in such a way. This experience of illness felt to be punishment reenacts the childhood experience that if one is good one is rewarded but if one is bad one is punished.

Hierarchy of Body Parts

Another facet affecting the patient's attitude toward illness has to do with the perceived hierarchy of body parts. The importance of various organs to any one individual is determined by both cultural and idiosyncratic issues. Thus, it is fairly universal that the heart and the brain are on the top of any list. It is obvious that surgery on the heart appears to the patient to be more dramatic than surgery on the liver although both organs are vital. When heart transplants were first done, accounts of the procedure filled the front pages of most newspapers worldwide. At the same time, liver transplants were being conducted and although these are technically more difficult than the heart procedures, they received little or no notice. Organs such as the pancreas or adrenal, may be relatively silent in the patient's psyche. The anxiety evoked by circumcision may be greater than that preceding splen-ectomy although the latter is obviously a more major procedure. For some women undergoing mastectomy, the loss of the breast may be at that time more difficult to endure than the awareness of having cancer. In performing breast surgery it must be borne in mind that the breast as representing feminity may be more important in some cultures, such as that of the United States, than in other countries, such as certain Asian nations, and the loss of a breast may therefore have a greater significance.

For some patients the organ or disease process may have a personal meaning far different from that experienced by another patient. For example, two men may be given the diagnosis of diabetes mellitus. One may have had a diabetic father who experienced shocks and comas, diabetic neuropathies and retinopathies, blindness, and amputations. The other may have had a diabetic father whose disease was controlled by diet and who lived into his nineties. While both men may be given the same diagnosis, it is certain that their reactions to the doctor's words will be different. In the same way, a person who has been told that she needs an appendectomy may become anxious out of proportion if someone close to her has had a disastrous result following a similar procedure. Thus, a patient's own personal history may determine the reaction to the surgery.

Personal History

A young woman with a long history of duodenal ulcer required surgery for pyloric stenosis but at the last minute she became anxious and refused surgery. The psychiatrist took another medical history and learned that although she had told the surgeon that her father had died of leukemia, in reality he had died immediately after an operation for carcinoma of the stomach. It was clear that the cause of the father's death given to the surgeon was an attempt on her part to dissociate her own illness from his and she expected to die in the same way, since she thought that she too must have carcinoma. When this was discussed and her medical condition clearly elucidated, her anxiety abated and she agreed to the operation.

It is hard to imagine that patients can come to surgery without being profoundly affected by previous experiences both in their own lives and in the lives of close members of the family and friends. Thus, the explanation for some unexpected reactions on the part of patients to suggested procedures can be sought only in the history of both themselves and their loved ones. While this is a rather obvious conclusion, it is striking how frequently this is neglected in the care of our patients. All too often these personal issues are left unaddressed and the patient is treated with drugs in an attempt to alleviate anxiety or depression.

A liaison psychiatrist was asked to see a 58-year-old housewife who was profoundly depressed on admission for a vascular procedure. Her history revealed that she had been seriously depressed over the past 10 years and had been treated with antidepressants. The drugs had been successful in alleviating her symptoms and after several months her doctor had discontinued the medication. Her depressive symptoms shortly returned and again she was medicated. When the symptoms diminished, she herself decided to discontinue the drug. Once more her symptoms returned. This pattern was frequently repeated over the next 10 years. During the psychiatric interview the patient revealed that no one had ever taken a history of the depression, but her doctors had assumed that it was in reaction to a colostomy she had had for colon cancer at the time her depression began. However, she was very specific in her dating the onset of her depression to the fourth postoperative day when she awoke in the ICU feeling dejected and suicidal. The fact that she could specifically date the onset of the depression piqued the curiosity of the examiner and he learned that 20 years before, her mother had had the same surgery. The patient was the same age as her mother at the time of her operation. On the third postoperative day, her mother had suddenly died. The patient fully expected to follow in her mother's footsteps and was surprised to wake up on the fourth postoperative day. A discussion of her guilt feelings about her survival led to a rapid and complete disappearance of her depressive symptoms. Follow-up over a two-year period showed no return of the depression and no need for medication.

In this case, a knowledge of the patient's past history allowed her to be treated for the root cause of her difficulty rather than via the alleviation of her symptoms with medication. Paradoxical depressions of this sort will be discussed later in this chapter in the section on postoperative reactions.

The three periods for a surgical patient—preoperative, intraoperative, and postoperative—present different psychological problems for the patient as well as for the physician. These three periods are discussed next.

PREOPERATIVE

From the patient's perspective, there is no such thing as "minor" surgery. One can even think of this as a technical surgical term. The patient's fear of mutilation and death is also matched by the threat of exploration inherent in any surgical (and even medical or laboratory) procedure. In addition, the patient's fantasy of risk concerning anesthesia and surgery usually far exceeds the realistic dangers involved. Yet the patient does not usually share his or her concerns with the physician. Indeed, some patients who seem calm and contained clinically, may reveal a level of anxiety close to psychosis when psychological tests are performed (Meyer, Brown, Levine, 1955). In addition, patients may be reluctant to share their anxieties with their surgeons lest the surgeons take their worries as an indication of lack of confidence in the physicians' operative skills.

In elective procedures, patients may find themselves subject to a mounting level of anxiety over a number of days only to have the anxiety abate on the day prior to surgery as the mechanism of denial effectively wards off anxiety. At times we hear surgeons suggest that they would worry about a patient who is not anxious preoperatively, yet one can question this, since we know that patients who are not anxious require less anesthetic agent and seem to face the ordeal with greater equanimity and therefore a better physiological situation. That this denial is more than one of cosmetic appearance is attested to by the fact that preoperative cardiac surgery patients in general appear less anxious than those facing general surgery. The same psychologist who discovered a high degree of anxiety in preoperative patients before general surgery studied the same psychological tests pre- and postoperatively in cardiac patients and found that the level of anxiety preoperatively was much lower in most patients than in the postoperative state, unlike what was seen in the patients in his 1955 study. This suggests that the greater the danger, as perceived by the patient, the greater may be the denial (Brown & Blacher, unpublished data).

Informed Consent

The patient is asked to give permission for the surgery and it is sometimes assumed that the explanation, at times a lengthy one, given by the surgeon preoperatively informs the patient sufficiently so that he or she may make a valid judgment. One must wonder about this, since despite the most careful explanation of the procedure, the anxiety of the patient often precludes the possibility of his understanding. For example, after a detailed explanation by the surgeon of a heart precedure, it is not uncommon for a patient to ask the psychiatrist in a routine interview a question such as, "When they take my heart out during the operation, will they keep it in the same room as my body?" In a study of patients' reactions to valve surgery, the surgeon described in detail and with the use of a model how he would remove the old valve and replace it. Later, in discussing the procedure, over 50 percent of the patients insisted that their hearts had not been opened (Blacher, 1971). Merav and Robinson (1976) made a similar observation when they tape-recorded the description of the procedure and their examination of the patient and then queried the patient four to six months later as to what the patient had been told. Although the consultation lasted up to 45 minutes, most patients described an exceedingly brief contact with no information exchanged. Often those patients who were most adamant in what they insisted had not been told were the ones who had been given the most detailed explanation. It would certainly seem that in this situation the greater the fantasied danger the greater the anxiety and therefore the greater the difficulty in understanding what the physician says.

Cancellation of Surgery

It is not unusual on a busy surgical service for operations of an elective nature to be canceled and rescheduled, especially when emergencies involving other patients occur. If his own medical condition, such as a skin rash, intercurrent infection, or an abnormal laboratory finding interferes with his scheduled procedure, the patient may be disappointed but his cognitive understanding helps to ease the letdown which occurs. His is an ambivalent situation. He fears the surgery but has prepared himself for it and thus is disappointed. However, when another patient's necessity causes cancellation of his operation, the patient's reaction may be quite strong. He has gone through the process of psychologically preparing himself for the ordeal, and must now begin his preparation anew. He is able to understand the *necessity* for performing an emergency operation in place of his own elective one, but cannot really be expected to consider any case as more important than his own. A depression-prone man has been witnessed to go into a suicidal depression when told by an unthinking house officer "we have to cancel your operation because a more serious case was just admitted." The patient is in a serious conflict; on the one hand he recognizes other peoples' needs, but on the other hand, in his partly regressed situation he is unable to empathize with anyone else. Nor should it be expected that he empathize with others, since it is understandable that his narcissistic regression causes him to focus on his own problems at such a time. Needless to say, old sibling rivalry issues may intensify this reaction. The patient's natural response is to feel a sense of outrage at the medical staff. However, he feels particularly vulnerable, being angry at the very people on whom he counts to save his life. In addition, his partially regressed state makes him feel that even *thoughts* of anger will be known by his attendants. Under these circumstances, it is not unusual for the patient then to become depressed. It is remarkably therapeutic for such patients to be told that their anger is understandable and even expectable, and therefore completely safe. When this is discussed with a patient, it is usual for the depression to lift immediately.

Preoperative Anxiety

It is very clear that the anxiety of patients need bear no relationship to what their physicians think is the seriousness of the condition. A patient's optimism may be boundless in the face of a doleful prognosis or the patient may feel a minor procedure has ominous overtones. Clearly, the patient's fantasies about his condition have a greater significance than the realities as seen by the doctor. Thus in a way the patient may suffer from the physician's expertise, since the physician may assume that the patient shares his view of the situation. Sometimes the patient's personality may determine the atmosphere in a dramatic way.

A 75-year-old woman faced surgery for which she was told that there was a 15 percent risk of dying. Although she was quite clear mentally, she misinterpreted the surgeon's words and announced to a group of students who were interviewing her that "my chances of living are 15 percent." The interviewer remarked, "That seems terrible." To this the patient smiled and said, "Oh not at all. Two years ago I had an operation where I had only a 5% chance of surviving. These odds are three times better and I will make it, don't you worry." The patient did indeed sail through her surgery with no difficulty. Her bubbling optimism had clearly maintained her through many difficult times in her life.

Undue, overt anxiety should always cause the physician to wonder what the patient is *really* worried about. George Bernard Shaw's golden rule "Do not do unto others as you would that they should do unto you. Their tastes may not be the same" (Shaw, 1946) might be considered in our dealing with patients in such circumstances. Great tact is required in learning about the patient's fears, since opposing his feeling of being free to reveal his concerns to the physician are the perceived dangers of (1) questioning the knowledge and authority of the doctor, (2) appearing ignorant in the eyes of people whom he wants very much to respect him and therefore take care of him, and (3) being thought odd or even insane if he talks of his fantasies. Thus, the patient may have trouble expressing worries.

A 50-year-old woman was admitted for a lung biopsy after a routine x-ray revealed a suspicious mass. She was still mourning the death of an older sister a year before, a sister who had died of lung cancer and one on whom the patient had modeled her life. She had managed to follow the sister's example in her choice of spouse, the number of children she had had, and even in the choice of employment when the children had left home. As the day for surgery approached, she realized to her horror that it was scheduled for the very anniversary of her sister's death. She made a concerted effort to hide her growing fears, lest her physicians think her "silly and crazy." To her immense relief the surgery had to be postponed. She was finally able to tell of this fear only in the context of a postoperative depression, after *her* biopsy revealed a benign condition.

The physician stands *in loco parentis* with a patient who wants to appear good. The patient wants to be admired and loved and thus treated well and cured. The physician is handled with kid gloves and despite the doctor's wish that the patient tell him about his anxieties, the patient may be loath to do so lest the physician lose respect for him. This problem requires that the physician not only be sensitive, but to a degree be able to put himself in the position of the patient, to think like a patient rather than as a medical professional.

One irrational fear that patients are reluctant to discuss with the physician is the superstitution that bad things happen in threes. While other super-stitions are not unusual, this one is met with most frequently (Blacher, 1983). Thus, a patient who has had two previous surgeries may be worried that "the third strike means you're out." If two members of his immediate family have died in the recent past, he may fear that he will be the third. The ability to talk about this without ridicule by the medical staff allows the patient to feel more comfortable.

ANESTHESIA AND THE INTRAOPERATIVE PERIOD

The patient facing surgery is put into the position of being damned if he does and damned if he doesn't. He looks for anesthesia to prevent pain and provide him with oblivion during the procedure. Yet ironically he also fears the anesthesia. At the very least he fears loss of control involved in putting himself in the hands of a total stranger who will have the power of life and death over him. He may even equate imposed sleeping with dying. Telling a youngster that he will be "put to sleep during surgery" would hardly seem reassuring if that youngster has had a pet sent to the veterinarian for just such an act. In addition, many patients are afraid that with the loss of control, as they are being anesthetized, they will reveal all sorts of secrets. Although this does not occur, it is frequently a source of worry to the patient and should be addressed by the physician if he suspects such a concern.

Here too, the patient suffers from the physician's competence. There is a natural tendency to assume that what is commonplace for us is commonplace for others, and since medical procedures are an everyday occurrence in the hospital, it is easy to forget that surgical situations are unique and therefore frightening for the patient. Usually, the fantasy of what is to happen is worse than reality and thus an open explanation may actually be anxiety-relieving to the average person. The anesthesiologist is in a unique position in dealing with the perioperative experience, since the care of the patient is entrusted to him before, during, and immediately after the operation. The patient usually has an opportunity to have contact with the surgeon as he undergoes the initial physical examination. He can then feel himself in good hands and even idealize the doctor. However, since it is the anesthesiologist who meets him and puts him to sleep in the operating room a preoperative visit with the anesthesiologist who will be present at the induction usually has a calming effect. Patients visited beforehand come to the operating theater calm, even if not sedated. Those who are given medication in lieu of a visit by the anesthesiologist may come to the operating room anxious and sedated and require more anesthetic agent than their visited counterparts (Egbert, Battit, Turndorf, & Beecher, 1963).

Modern surgery had its origin with the introduction of general anesthesia in 1846. With patients having surgery without pain, the surgeon could focus on technique rather than speed, knowing that the patient would be insensible during the procedure. Prior to general anesthesia, the patients would be restrained and traumatized (Guerra, 1980). Prior to the use of anesthesia, reviews of mortality during surgery suggested that pain and the fear of pain were among the most common causes of death (Whitby, 1975).

While the older anesthetic agents, such as ether and chloroform, fairly consistently provided analgesia and amnesia, they also presented problems in toxicity. Ether induction caused a phase of excitement, with the patient feeling suffocated. It was not unusual during this time for him to have an out-of-body experience. When curare was introduced in 1942 (Griffith & Johnson, 1942), muscular relaxation was effected and it was then possible to maintain patients relaxed with a lower depth of anesthesia. This was accompanied, however, by an increased difficulty in monitoring the level of consciousness. It was assumed with older anesthestic agents that when the patient was unconscious no pain was experienced. The newer drugs allowed the patient to awaken and yet be totally paralyzed (Scott, 1972). The technique of using newer intravenous agents along with muscle relaxants, a technique called "balanced anesthesia," allowed for greater physiologic control during anesthesia and caused fewer toxic reactions. However, the anesthesiologist had then to keep in mind the possibility of the patient's awakening and being unable to move because of the relaxant. Starting in 1950, reports began to appear describing the experience of awakening under these circumstances (Winterbottom, 1950).

A study to evaluate such reactions was undertaken with relatively light anesthesia (Levinson, 1965). The results suggested that patients were able to respond to noxious verbal stimuli despite apparent unconsciousness during a dental procedure. In an attempt to replicate the study, but using deeper anesthesia in major surgery, we were able to recover such a stimulus. In the midst of the operation, the anesthesiologist turned off his machine for a few seconds and announced in a loud voice "The patient is turning blue; we have to stop the operation." Later the patient was hypnotized and brought back to the operative time and was then able to account in exact detail what was said (Blacher, Winkelstein & Meyer, unpublished data). Since we found this experiment too inhumane to continue, we tried benign stimuli instead and were unsuccessful in attempts at recovering them. We wondered whether patients might register stimuli only when such stimuli had an important significance. Recall under general anesthesia might be thought of as only theoretically upsetting, but we have seen a series of patients (Meyer & Blacher, 1961; Blacher, 1975, 1984) who awakened from light anesthesia during surgery while paralyzed by succinylcholine. These patients had a postoperative traumatic neurosis marked by (1) repetitive nightmares usually of poorly disguised versions of an operative situation, (2) anxiety and irritability, (3) a preoccupation with death, and (4) a concern with sanity that made them reluctant to discuss their symptoms. They were confused as to whether they had actually awakened during surgery, and were cured of their symptoms by the simple explanation that they had indeed been awake. During this (usually) brief time that the patient is awake, he feels that something must have gone terribly wrong, for why else would he be awake? The symptoms resemble those seen following other acute psychic traumata. Since patients can undergo surgery while completely awake, as in local or spinal anesthesia, it is clearly not the fact of awareness itself that is the important issue; rather it seems the sense of passively experiencing an event over which one has no control but where the feeling is that things have somehow gone awry that is traumatic. Patients are unable to call for help and since they are in a somewhat obtunded state they question whether what they experienced could even possibly have taken place. The patient who is wide awake may suffer a great deal during the procedure but seems to have fewer traumatic symptoms afterwards, perhaps because there is no question that the event actually occurred. Indeed, patients who are anesthetized with large doses of morphine as the sole anesthetic for cardiac surgery do not suffer postoperatively. It is customary for the anesthesiologist, who recognizes that the patient is awake, to talk constantly to the patient in a reassuring manner (Lowenstein, Hallowell, Levine, Daggett, Austen, & Lever 1969).

A few case histories will illustrate this syndrome:

Case 1

A 25-year-old hospital secretary underwent a major abdominal procedure under intravenous Pentothal and nitrous oxide anesthesia, supplemented by succinylcholine. She had been followed by a liaison psychiatrist through a series of illnesses and was seen frequently during the hospitalization and it was noted that she had a general irritability about which she refused to talk. However, on discharge she called for an appointment at the hospital and disclosed that she had been bothered by a recurrent nightly nightmare of hearing voices and seeing people floating over her all in an aura of blue. She felt she was choking and couldn't defend herself and the prominent feeling was that she was dead or dying, perhaps in heaven. She would then wake in terror and be unable to go back to sleep. Since the surgery, she was constantly preoccupied with death. She had not spoken of her symptoms in the hospital for fear that she would be considered insane, but now she felt overwhelmed. When it was suggested that she must have been awake during surgery, she began to connect the dream with her experience. She could identify all the people in her nightmare—masked and dressed in blue—and could recall her surgeon giving specific orders. The choking sensation had to do with the endotracheal tube. The night after her discussion she had the dream again, but instead of experiencing the usual terror, she laughed and went back to sleep. The nightmare never recurred afterward; her irritability disappeared, and she felt normal by the day after the talk. With this patient, it was clear that the nightmare had reproduced the actual events, but the patient had not connected the dreams with the experience. Such patients are typically relieved of their symptoms by confirming for them that their nightmares had actually occurred.

Case 2

A 43-year-old man after mitral valve replacement was noted to be irritable and anxious. He was unable to sleep at night and when questioned, revealed that he had a repetitive nightmare of being tied down and having some unknown people sticking things into him. When it was suggested that he had been awake during surgery, he seemed relieved and his symptoms disappeared.

Case 3

A 54-year-old man had an unusual type of repetitive dream following coronary artery bypass surgery. He had the usual symptoms but described a different nightmare every night. The common denominator in his dreams was that he was in some place where he desperately wanted to get out but could not do so. One night he dreamed of being in a large crowd being carried along into a dangerous situation and he was unable to extricate himself. The next night he was locked in a cell trying to escape. Although all the dreams were different, the general tone of desperately wanting to escape was present in all. He also responded when it was suggested that his symptoms resulted from his having been awake during the operation.

Case 4

A 48-year-old patient insisted that his dreams of being tied down and unable to move were related to a recollection of being sewn up at the time at the end of surgery. When the examiner suggested that it might have been a dream or his imagination, he adamantly insisted that he was sure he had been awake. When told that he *was* awake at the end of surgery, the patient seemed shocked and exclaimed "I was?" Despite his certainty, he was startled to have his observation confirmed.

The plaint of these patients was summed up well by Claude Bernard (1878) in discussing the effects of curare:

In all ages poetic fictions which seek to arouse our pity have presented us with sensitive beings locked in immobile bodies. Our imagination cannot conceive of anything more unhappy than beings provided with sensation, that is to say of being able to feel pleasure and pain, when they are deprived of the power to flee the one and yearn toward the other. The torture which the imaginations of poets has invented can be found produced in nature by the action of the American poison. We can even say that the fiction falls short of reality.

Thus, the symptoms, which closely resemble those seen after any severe, acute trauma, are an attempt to deal with this helpless state. The patient suffers with a sense of unreality—as noted, the patient can't quite believe that what was experienced could actually have occurred, and is reluctant to talk about it lest others consider him to be insane. This reluctance, seen even in a patient such as the first case, who was being followed by a psychiatrist, suggests that these episodes may actually occur more often than has been noted. The repetitive dreams can be seen as an attempt to master during sleep what was experienced as overwhelming during a state of being awake (Freud, 1920).

The implications of the possibility that the patient might hear what is said during surgery is clear. It would seem to behoove those in the operating theater to temper what they say. This is not a new idea. As long ago as 1914 Crile and Lower described their experience in eliminating all afferent stimuli in the perioperative situation. Their results were dramatic in showing improvement in the postoperative condition of their patients, including a lowered mortality rate.

Although the patient usually thinks of general anesthesia when confronting surgery, the method of choice may be local or spinal. However, these methods may also create certain problems for the patient. The postoperative anxiety from being immobilized by paralysis of the lower extremities is known to every anesthesiologist and yet the need to reassure the patient at this point is not always considered. The operating staff must also reflect on the fact that such patients are awake even when obtunded and they must not treat them as if they were deeply anesthetized.

Since the illness and the surgery intended to cure the condition are in the foreground, it is easy for the medical staff to forget that from the patient's point of view the anesthesia plays a prominent role in the hospital experience.

POSTOPERATIVE

The Immediate Postoperative Period

Since the patient is able to experience stimuli while under the influence of anesthesia, one would expect that this ability must also be present in the recovery room. Many medical personnel have felt that on awakening from surgery, patients are in a markedly obtunded state and not aware of their surroundings. Close observation suggests otherwise (Winkelstein, Blacher, & Meyer, 1965). Observations of patients who were seemingly out of contact revealed that they were, in general, easily aroused and interested in their medical conditions. When approached by strangers they would exhibit a clear sensorium but a remarkably casual attitude, apparently a manifestation of denial. When the patients' own physicians visited, they presented an entirely different picture, being clearly interested in knowing the outcome of the surgery and eager for assurance. Patients often wanted to know whether a condition was malignant, in order for them to begin coming to grips with the situation. The patients could recall in great detail the recovery room experience when asked about it several days later.

The Intensive Care Unit

Frequently patients who have had complicated surgery are sent to an intensive care unit (ICU). Here they are monitored and supervised very closely. The intensive care unit might be considered the epitome of ambivalence for the patient. Patients realize they are in the ICU because their lives are in danger and so they wish to be transferred to the regular part of the hospital; on the other hand, if their lives are in danger there can be no better place than the ICU. Transfer to a regular floor when improvement warrants it, may be accompanied by a great deal of anxiety.

The ICU is a strange environment for patients. They are surrounded by an array of devices which seem to be straight out of science fiction. These devices emit sounds and blink lights while the patient lies immobilized, with tubes and wires inserted in every natural orifice and into a number of artificially made orifices as well. Often patients are intubated and unable to speak and therefore unable to let their needs be known to the nurses. The immobilization of a patient is often not appreciated. At a time when it is fair to say that patients are struggling with massive anxiety about their condition and treatment, they are unable to take advantage of a technique that most people have available when under stress—namely, the use of movement to lower tension.

One might think of the reaction in a group of expectant fathers, to taking their coffee and cigarettes away and strapping them into beds. The experience of pain and anxiety and the inability to deal with them by usual coping mechanisms makes it understandable that the ICU experience may be remembered as a terrifying one.

It is not surprising that under these circumstances some patients react by a massive psychic withdrawal from reality into a psychosis. But *overt* psychotic reactions are not the rule. "ICU psychosis" is a catchy term but one which does not truly capture the essence of the problem, since it is not the ICU itself which is connected with psychosis but the type of illness and treatment which seem responsible for major reactions. The writer worked in a large ICU during the early days of such units where patients were treated after cardiac surgery, myocardial infarction, and lung surgery. The coronary and lung surgery patients were almost never psychotic, whereas almost all of the cardiac surgery patients had major psychic upheavals, despite the fact that they were in the same environment. Both the extent of the illness and the treatment seem to be more important in this respect than the environment itself despite the fact that the environment may be terrifying (Sgroi, Holland, & Marwit, 1968; Blacher, 1972). Sgroi, Holland, and Marwit found this to be true in their cases, where the rate of psychosis depended on the degree of illness rather than the location of the patient.

Both organic and psychological factors seem to work synergistically in creating emotional difficulties. The most common psychological reaction in ICUs is paranoia, sometimes to the extent of the patients defending themselves violently against the ministrations of the nurses, and thus disrupting the treatment. It is interesting to note that the paranoia—the feeling that the staff is trying to kill the patient—almost invariably involves only the nurses, rarely the physicians. This is not surprising if we consider that the paranoia is a projection of the rage that patients feel as a result of their treatment. In a regressed state because of their medical condition, they wish to be left alone. Like young children who do not appreciate the necessity for medical interventions, patients resent the fact that they are asked to move around, to breathe deeply, to get out of bed. They are subjected to frequent injections, tracheal suctioning, and other painful treatments. Under these circumstances patients find themselves enraged but are afraid of being angry at the very people they count on to maintain their lives. Because of the regression, patients feel even the thought of anger will be known by the nurses. Therefore, the only safe thing to do with the resentment is to project it. The theme becomes "I don't want to kill *you* because I am so angry at what you do; you want to kill *me*." Most of the time this paranoid episode is hidden (Blacher, 1972) and the patients may tell no one of their fear, not even members of their families. This is probably because they realize the psychotic nature of their feeling. Such hidden reactions may be more damaging than overt manifestations, since the latter are usually dealt with. The writer has seen patients who had such paranoid episodes, which they revealed only years later, having suffered in the interval with a feeling that since they had such a mental aberration in the past, they were always in imminent danger of having this psychotic episode recur.

A major contributing element to these paranoid episodes is the wish by the nursing staff to be liked and appreciated. Despite the fact that they know their ministrations are painful, they would like the patients to appreciate their efforts. After much work with nurses in the cardiac ICU, they have been able to use a different approach to the patient. They are able to let the patient know that *they* can appreciate that the natural human reaction to being poked and pushed is to feel resentful, and that they, the nurses, fully expect the patients to dislike the treatment. The theme becomes "You don't have to like it, you just have to take it." The patients feel that they have permission to be angry, and therefore the danger of being angry is diminished. Since the inauguration of this change, we have rarely seen episodes of paranoia in the ICU, although other surgical ICUs not using this technique report such cases (Blacher & Cleveland, 1979).

ORGANIC MENTAL DIFFICULTIES

Not uncommon after surgery are organic mental difficulties, ranging from agitated delirium to mild deficits ascertained only by testing. The causes for these changes are legion, ranging from reactions to analgesics, metabolic dysfunctions, and complications of surgery. Despite the patent organic background, the understanding and treatment of this condition, aside from correcting the underlying cause, is to a great degree psychologic.

In a sense, we do not see the organic dysfunction in the patients' behavior. What we do see is the psychological attempt to deal with the deficit. In addition, the content of the patients' productions may reveal what their anxiety is about. If one sits with a patient one knows very well, in the midst of delirious "gibberish," one realizes that one can understand much of what the patient is trying to say. To the person who does not know the inner life of the patient the verbal productions make no sense. Despite the underlying organic difficulty, how the patient deals with the deficit depends on a number of psychological factors. One can think of alcoholic intoxication as a paradigm. We know that the response to such a cerebral toxin is usually determined more by social demands and expectations than by the brain level of the drug. Thus, the person who is inebriated, when confronted by an emergency, may act in a fairly normal manner. We have observed that despite marked confusion in the midst of a delirium cardiac patients almost never attempt to touch their chest tubes, while gallbladder patients may attempt to remove their drains, indicating that despite the confusion the heart patients nevertheless are attempting to preserve their lives. Both in chronic and acute situations, patients with organic impairment rarely complain to the physician of their difficulty. Nevertheless, organically impaired patients respond emotionally to the loss of their brain function—a most frightening state for most patients. Delirious patients can be reassured that with medical care they will recover their minds and this comforting observation will often have a dramatically soothing and quieting effect even in patients who a minute before had insisted that there was nothing wrong with their mentation. This reassurance, along with an attempt to keep the environment as stable as possible, for example, the presence of the same nurses and members of the family if feasible and the use of a night light so there are visual clues rather than the confusion of darkness and ominous-seeming shadows, all should be employed in the patients' treatment. Careful explanation of all procedures may be very useful.

Past history may determine the patients' reactions and compound the confusion.

A 50-year-old woman with a portacaval shunt developed delirium after her surgery and attempted to remove her intravenous lines and her drains. She was restrained by wrist straps but this caused a marked increase in her agitation. An elder sister reported that as a young child the patient had been tied into bed while her mother went out of the house. The restraints obviously had rekindled a memory of this early distressing experience. While she could not be trusted with the free use of her hands, she was given calm and repeated explanations for the restraint and this resulted in a striking lessening of her excitement.

The mental state of such a patient makes it difficult for her to judge reality correctly and thus increases her anxiety to a major degree. This anxiety, in turn, makes the patient's ability to judge even worse and so there is a vicious circle that must be broken at some point. It must be remembered that acute delirium may signal a worsening of the patient's medical condition, for example, the development of a major fever or hyperglycemia or hypoxia (Titchener, Zwerling, Gottschalk, Levine, Culbertson, Cohen, & Silver, 1956).

It is surprising how seldom one sees dramatic psychological reactions following general surgery. Although certain situations may show a high rate of overt psychosis (heart surgery in its earlier years), most patients handle their postoperative situation well. Patients who have had prior psychosis rarely decompensate. Chronic schizophrenics may even be model patients, and we have seen chronically hallucinatory patients undergo surgery with no difficulty. It is not uncommon for such patients' mental states to be known only to their psychiatric consultants with no overt evidence apparent to their other medical attendants. Such patients may be somewhat withdrawn and undemanding and create no problem. In the rare instance of a vulnerable patient having an outbreak of an underlying psychosis when undergoing the stress of surgery, the treatment is usually the same as it is for any other patient on a psychiatric service. The rate of postoperative psychosis varies in different studies from less than 1 percent (Knox, 1961) in a study where statistics were gleaned from charts of patients who required psychiatric hospitalization, up to 22 percent (Titchener, Zwerling, Gottschalk, Levine, Culbertson, Cohen, & Silver, 1956) in a study where the patient population was interviewed by psychiatrists. The same variation has been noted in studies of heart surgery (Kornfeld, Zimberg, & Malm, 1965; Blacher, 1972).

Most psychological problems seen postoperatively are more subtle and may present as medical difficulties rather than purely psychological states. For example, this is seen when depressions are manifested by anorexia, a difficulty in being mobilized and an inability to follow simple medical regimens. These depressive symptoms may create a medical emergency, since they often do not respond to medical efforts and may lead to sequelae such as thrombophlebitis, pneumonia, poor wound healing, or decubitus ulcers.

A common source of anxiety is the varying degree of organic mental impairment that patients may experience following surgery. This is especially true for heart patients but is certainly seen in other patients undergoing general anesthesia and the use of consciousness-clouding medications. Patients are reluctant to reveal the impairment or the fact that they have had the impairment in the recent past. They are afraid that their physicians will think they are insane, or in the case of older patients, that they will be considered senile. At times the use of denial will make patients unable to see the dysfunction but usually their awareness is quite conscious. When the examiner is able to demonstrate the deficit to the patient, by means of simple mental testing, he is then able to reassure the patient that this a transient phenomenon. What the patient worries about is not the episode itself but its implications for the future, namely senility or a sense of having a sword hanging over one's head that might fall again at any moment. Permanent brain damage, in our experience, is rare, unless there is a major cerebral insult in the perioperative period.

DEPRESSIONS AND PSEUDODEPRESSIONS

Many of the depressive reactions seen following surgery are, in reality, not depressions at all from the dynamic point of view, but rather are closely akin to mourning states. Such reactions commonly occur following mutilating operations and even after the loss of internal organs. The patient reacts with a sense of loss to the removal of a body part (a limb or a breast), to the loss of a function (the loss of a sensory modality as in blindness, or deafness, or the use of limbs as in paralysis), or to the loss of a sense of bodily integrity (the removal of an organ which has a strong psychic meaning). The danger in having such reactions classified as depression has to do with the treatment on the part of the medical staff. Certainly, the patients' medical attendants feel terrible in the face of a woman weeping after a mastectomy and at times, in order to make themselves feel better, they will try to cheer her up by telling her that she is *lucky* because the pathology report showed that the nodes were negative. This may be the equivalent of telling a woman who has just lost a child in a fire that she should feel lucky that her other children were saved. Cases of loss such as this should be considered equivalent to the loss of a love object and the patient should be treated with a warm, sympathetic, and supportive attitude. Brief reactions should certainly not be *interpreted*, but rather allowed to run their course. Usually within a week or two the patient is noted to be more cheerful. If the depressive symptoms continue, a further explanation may be considered.

The cause of a true depressive reaction may be more difficult to ascertain—certainly its cause may be less obvious but usually can be discovered in an interview when one is alert to dynamic issues. A true depression can usually be differentiated from a grief reaction by the latter's appropriateness in response to a loss and by the depressive person's self-critical attitude—in other words, guilt. At times this may even involve suicidal thoughts. The grief stricken patient's attitude is: "Without the part of me that I have lost the world is terrible, although I, myself, am all right." The depressive patient feels that the world is all right, but "I, myself, am worthless." Grief reactions are almost invariably direct and open. As noted, depressions may present as difficulties in medical management.

Depressions

While depressions after surgery are not as common as grief reactions, they nevertheless occur and, as mentioned, may create medical difficulties for the patient. They range in magnitude from mild, fleeting feelings lasting a few hours or a day or two to profound and even suicidal affects, such as described previously in the woman with colonic cancer. What is important in the understanding, and therefore in the treatment of postoperative depressions, is the realization that they do not spring spontaneously from the surgical incision. They always have a meaning, and if one can understand this meaning the treatment is often direct. The use of antidepressant medication, rather than the exploration of psychological difficulties, may be unfortunate for several reasons. First, it takes a long time to be effective, and second, its use may allow the physician and patient to avoid treating the underlying problem that may act as a focus of difficulty in the years to come.

The most common cause of depression appearing a few days after a surgical procedure is survivor guilt. This was illustrated by the woman with colonic cancer. It is not uncommon on the third day following coronary bypass surgery, when the patient has many of his life support systems removed and realizes that he will now survive on his own, for him to go into a profound depression. Invariably, these patients give a history of other members of the family who have died of heart disease at an age younger than they are at present. Some patients may be the only surviving members of families whose genetic background resulted in coronary artery disease. Strikingly, these patients reveal that they had not expected to survive the operation, and when they do realize that they will live they have a paradoxical depression rather than a great sense of relief. This reaction is reminiscent of Freud's patients who were "wrecked by success" (Freud, 1916), that is, people who have a depression initiated not by loss but rather by a gain in prestige, position, or material possessions.

A 46-year-old man entered the hospital for biopsy of a suspicious-looking lymph node in his neck. A resection was done and several days later the surgeon was able to report to the patient the good news that the lesion was totally benign. An hour later, the patient was found to be markedly depressed with suicidal ruminations. His history revealed that two years before, his older brother, an idol of his from childhood, had died of sarcoma, after the initial diagnosis had been made by cervical node biopsy. He had assumed that his lesion would be the same, and from the time of the surgeon's report, he had thought of nothing but this brother as he became more and more depressed.

This man, like most of the people who become depressed postoperatively, had never suffered depression before and had functioned well. Exploration of these patients (Blacher, 1978) reveals that the dynamics have to do with what can be called a "quantitative view" of death. This view, shared by many people in our culture, holds that nature demands a certain number of deaths, and if one person dies another can be spared.

This was evident in wartime when two men would share a foxhole and one was killed by a bomb. The survivor would often become depressed and would reveal the general theme of "as long as one of us *had* to die, I am glad it wasn't me." However, what this meant to the patient was that he was glad that his buddy, whom he loved, had died "instead of me." For the soldier, his buddy was like a brother, and death could revive old ambivalent death wishes toward siblings. Treatment of these patients consists of pointing out that the depression is paradoxical, since one would expect that someone who hadn't thought he would live through surgery would feel like celebrating his survival rather than being depressed. "But how can you feel like celebrating when someone you love wasn't able to have a chance to live the way you have?" It can then be pointed out that the patient's living and the loved one's death had no connection, since the patient would have lived even if the other person also lived. The result of this intervention is usually a rapid relief of the depressive symptoms sometimes in a matter of minutes. One may wonder why such a simple statement is effective in these cases. The explanation probably lies in a number of factors: (1) the interviewer lends his superego to the patient and assures him that it is all right to be glad and (2) the interpretation has the quality of an "inexact interpretation" as formulated by Glover (1955). In these cases, the patient seizes on an interpretation as complete and therefore avoids confronting a more anxiety-provoking fantasy than the one presented. Thus, the thought of unconscious death wishes for the sibling are never approached. Also important is the fact that these patients feel guilty for unconscious thoughts rather than for having done anything harmful to anyone. Even the distance between the patient's recovery and his loved one's death makes it possible for him to dissociate the two. The fact that these patients have functioned well before suggests that they are helped by a relatively intact psychic apparatus to start with, rather than an excessively punishing superego.

On occasion, a surgeon may call on the psychiatrist for help in a similar type of depression, but one seen before any surgery is contemplated.

A 63-year-old factory worker came to the surgeon who had operated on him many years before, and who had saved his life with a dramatic pioneer procedure. He insisted that he now required another heroic effort because of increasing pains in his right arm and shoulder for the past month. Since the surgeon could find no major pathology, he requested a psychiatric consultation. The patient was the oldest son in an old-fashioned Italian family. When his parents had died, the patient had been in his twenties. He had assumed the role of patriarch and had taken his responsibilities seriously. A year prior to his calling the surgeon, he had buried his younger brother who had died of cancer involving his right arm and shoulder. He cried bitterly as he spoke of his feelings "It should have been me instead of him!" Treatment along the lines outlined previously were successful in relieving him of his symptoms.

Later Depressions

When patients are depressed at a later stage in their recovery it is often useful for the physician to wonder what they might be angry about, and such a question is frequently answered in an obvious way. For example, patients who develop wound infections or other complications will commonly become depressed. Those in whom a surgical procedure has been unsuccessful as in certain orthopedic cases or in recurrent cancer may find themselves in the same position. They feel in an untenable emotional conflict. They are angry that their physicians have let them down but are not able to accept this since (1) they may genuinely like their doctors and (2) they fear that even the thought of anger will stimulate a like response from their medical attendants and diminish their doctors efforts to rescue them. The anger is turned on themselves and is seen clinically as a depression. In this situation, treatment is directed at giving patients permission to feel angry by the consultant's suggesting that he would understand that the natural human reaction in this circumstance is to react in just that manner. The feeling of safety that patients have in experiencing their own resentment parallels the dealing with paranoia in the ICU. In the more regressed patients, anger seems to be projected; later in the recovery, it is turned on the self.

Other psychological reactions will be described in the following chapters. These will relate to the specific situations involved in specialized types of surgery.

REFERENCES

Bernard, C. (1878). *La Science Internationale*. Paris: Bailliere.

Blacher, R. S. (1971). Open heart surgery—The patient's point of view. *Mount Sinai Journal of Medicine, 38; 74.*

Blacher, R. S. (1972). The hidden psychosis of open heart surgery with a note on the sense of awe. *Journal of the American Medical Association, 222;* 305.

Blacher, R. S. (1975). On awakening paralyzed during surgery: A syndrome of traumatic neurosis, *Journal of American Medical Association, 234,* 67–68.

Blacher, R. S. (1978). Paradoxical depression after heart surgery: A form of survivor syndrome. *Psychoanalytic Quarterly, 47;* 267.

Blacher, R. S. (1983). Clusters of disaster: Superstition and the psychiatrist. *General Hospital Psychiatry, 5;* 279.

Blacher, R. S. (1984). Awareness during surgery (Editorial). *Journal of Anesthesiology, 61;* 1.

Blacher, R. S. and Cleveland, R. J. (1979). Heart surgery, *Journal of the American Medical Association, 242;* 2463.

Blacher, R. S., Winkelstein, C., & Meyer, B. C. Unpublished data.

Brown, F., & Blacher, R. S., Unpublished data.

Crile, A. W., Lower, W. E. (1914). *Anoci-Association.* Philadelphia: Saunders.

Egbert, L. D., Battit, G. E., Turndorf, H., & Beecher, H. K., (1963). The value of the preoperative visit by an anesthetist. A study of doctor-patient rapport. *Journal of the American Medical Association, 185;* 553.

Freud, S. (1916). Some character-types met with in psycho-analytic work. *Standard Edition* (Vol. 14, p. 311). London: Hogarth.

Freud, S. (1920). *Beyond the Pleasure Principle* (Vol. 18, p. 32). London: Hogarth Press.

Glover, E. (1955). *The Technique of Psycho-Analysis.* New York: International University Press.

Griffith, H. R., Johnson, G. E. (1942). Use of curare in general anesthesia. *Anesthesiology, 3;* 418–420.

Guerra, F. (1980). Awareness under general anesthesia. In F. Guerra, and J. A. Aldrete (Eds.), *Emotional and Psychological Responses to Anesthesia and Surgery (pp. 1-8).* New York: Grune & Stratton.

Knox, S. J. (1961). Severe psychiatric disturbances in the post- operative period — a five year survey of Belfast hospitals. *Journal of Mental Science, 107;* 1078.

Kornfeld, D. S., Zimberg, S., & Malm, J. R. (1965). Psychiatric complications of open-heart surgery. *New England Journal of Medicine, 273;* 287–292.

Levinson, B. W. (1965). States of awareness during general anesthesia. *British Journal of Anaesthesiology, 37;* 544.

Lowenstein, E., Hallowell, P., Levine, F. H., Daggett, W. M., Austen, W. G., & Lever, M. B. (1969). Cardiovascular response to large doses of intravenous morphine in man. *New England Journal of Medicine, 281;* 1389–1393.

Merav, A., & Robinson, G. (1976). Informed consent: Recalled by patients tested postoperatively. *Annals of Thoracic Surgery, 22;* 209.

Meyer, B. C., Blacher, R. S. (1961). A traumatic neurotic reaction induced by succinylcholine chloride. *New York State Journal of Medicine, 61;* 1255.

Meyer, B. C., Brown, F., & Levine, A. (1955). Observations of the house-tree-person drawing test before and after surgery. *Psychosomatic Medicine 17; 428.*

Scott, D. L. (1972). Awareness during general anesthesia. *Canadian Anaesth. Society Journal, 19;* 173–183.

Sgroi, S., Holland, J., & Marwit, S. J. (1968 March). *Psychological reactions to catastrophic illness.* Read before the annual meeting of the American Psychosomatic Society, Boston.

Shaw, G. B. (1946). Maxims for revolutionaries, in *Man and superman*, in *Selected Plays*. New York; Dodd, Mead.

Titchener, J. L., Zwerling, 1., Gottschalk, L., Levine, M., Culbertson, W., Cohen, S., & Silver, H. (1956). Psychosis in surgical patients. *Surgery, Gynecology & Obstetrics*, 102:59.

Whitby, J. D. (1975). Death during operation. *British Journal of Anaesthesiology, 47;* 408.

Winkelstein, C., Blacher, R. S., & Meyer, B. C. (1965). Psychiatric observation on surgical patients in recovery room. *New York State Journal of Medicine, 65;* 865.

Winterbottom, E. H. (1950). Insufficient anesthesia. *British Medical Journal, 1;* 247–248.

— CHAPTER TWO —

When Children
Have Surgery

JUDITH ELLEN ROBINSON, M.D.

Surgical procedures performed on children are events of great psychological significance. The fear and distrust that young patients have of doctors, hospitals, anesthesia, and surgery have been compellingly described in classical articles by Pearson (1941), Jackson (1942), Jessner and Kaplan (1949), and Coleman (1950). Behavioral changes have been documented in children who have undergone surgical procedures (Levy, 1945), even "minor" operations such as tonsillectomy (Jessner, Blom, & Waldfogel, 1952). The longlasting psychological effects of surgeries performed in childhood have been noted by psychoanalysts working with adult patients (Deutsch, 1942; Miller, 1951; Lipton, 1962). The purpose of this chapter is to review the current concepts of the psychological consequences of surgery in childhood and to relate these consequences to the age and developmental level of the child at the time of surgery, his life experiences and personality, relationships with parents, and to the specific medical condition under treatment.

AGE-RELATED REACTIONS

The Young Child

Unless there is severe physical pain, the stress of hospitalization for the young child derives from separation from parents. Among infants under six months of age, disorganization in the caretaking routine constitutes the major stress, whereas for older infants, loss of a specific caretaker predominates. Infants who have lengthy hospitalizations without visits from their family and without adequate holding and cuddling become depressed. They may "fail to thrive" despite excellent medical care. In extreme instances, infants may stop eating, may weaken and even die as a result of emotional deprivation.

For the toddler, as for the infant, separation from parents is a major problem. Indeed, this may so color the child's appreciation of the illness that suffering originating from without as opposed to from within the body cannot be distinguished (Freud, 1952). Not surprisingly, this reaction is exacerbated when the parents are themselves wrought with anxiety. The response of toddlers to prolonged separation, unlike that of infants, demonstrates the sequence of protest, despair, and detachment documented by Robertson (1958). When reunited with their parents, toddlers have difficulty reestablishing the former relationship with the caretakers whom they see as having deserted them.

Toddlers view their parents as omnipotent. Hence, they see their illness as a failure of their parents to protect them. This is particularly so in the case of children undergoing elective surgery who feel well before they enter the hospital and are unable to understand why they need an operation. These children see their parents' failure as a deliberate betrayal, abandonment, or punishment. The child may become angry, disappointed, and withdrawn. He may decathect his surroundings and focus all his energy on the preservation of life. The result may be a hypochondriacal child difficult to visit and to care for. Parents may respond with feelings of helplessness, anger, or guilt and may themselves withdraw in frustration, thereby reinforcing the child's feelings of abandonment.

Another set of problems arises from the fact that toddlers are striving to attain many new autonomous functions. In the hospital, they are asked to renounce these accomplishments and again be treated as babies. They may surrender developmental milestones, especially those which have been gained recently and are held tenuously. The loss is usually temporary; however, if the hospitalization is lengthy or traumatic, a current developmental task may cause particular conflicts with longlasting consequences.

Preschool and Early School Age

In the preschool and early school-age child, issues of separation and regression continue. Children of this age may have even more conflicts than younger children over enforced regression. While toddlers, not far removed from the time they enjoyed their mother's total loving care, may enjoy permission to be babies again (Bergman, 1945), older children often see enforced regression as giving in to infantile helplessness. They are threatened by castration anxiety, and boys may feel the stir of passive feminine longings. Children who struggle forcefully against these feelings tend to be noncompliant and difficult to manage.

In addition to the problems of separation and regression, preschool and early school-age children, now in the pre-Oedipal and Oedipal stages of development, worry a great deal about operations and bodily intrusions. They have multiple, often magical, fears about their illnesses, focusing on mutilation and castration. Frequently they see their illness as a punishment for certain thoughts or deeds, especially Oedipal transgressions. Most children of this age, whether they have diabetes, rheumatic fever, or chicken pox, have some feeling that they are responsible for what has happened to them. Beverly (1936) showed that 90 percent of the sick children interviewed stated they became ill "because they were bad." Eighty-five percent of the children with diabetes attributed their illness to "eating too much sugar," and 90 percent of the cardiac patients felt that they fell ill because they "ran too much." When children are involved in an accident in which they have violated some rule, for example, crossing the street without looking both ways or taking some medication they were not supposed to have taken, their sense of responsibility and guilt is heightened. In a world haunted by mother's warnings that failure to wear boots brings on a cold and eating too much candy brings on a stomach ache, it is not hard to understand why a sick child feels guilty and frightened and how hospitalization, with its separation from parents, restrictions, and painful procedures, confirms the child's worst suspicions of retribution. Many young children who are observed on the ward placidly accepting a painful procedure have given in to this fantasy and resigned themselves to whatever may come. Some children who are troubled by these guilty feelings project them onto others. These children are angry and rebellious with their parents and the staff (Freud, 1952). The following case illustrates some of the issues for a child of this age group.

Kevin had ulcerative colitis diagnosed when he was six. His disease was difficult to control and after two admissions to the ICU it was decided that he needed to have a colectomy. Prior to his surgery he was referred for psychotherapy. His doctors were concerned that he was unusually troubled by his disease and that without psychiatric intervention his adjustment to an ileostomy would be poor. In therapy, it became clear that he couldn't understand why he had ulcerative colitis but his brothers and sisters were unaffected. He couldn't understand that having ulcerative colitis had not to do with being "bad" or "good." This was complicated by the fact that he was "bad" a lot more often than he was "good." He couldn't understand that although he might improve his behavior and ask God to help, his illness was intractable and his surgery inevitable. He was angry, he hated himself, his parents, and he tried to pretend that he really wasn't sick by lying about his abdominal pain and his diarrhea.

With the help of psychotherapy, he began to see his illness as separate from his feelings and actions. His sense of guilt and responsibility diminished. He showed significant improvement, both in his self-esteem and in his adaptation to his illness.

As cognitive development proceeds, children's understanding of illness changes. Between 6 and 10 years of age, children begin to acquire a capacity for abstract reasoning and begin to grasp the causation of illness in a less personalized way. They are able to conceptualize medical conditions, such as diabetes and leukemia, which lack external stigmata. They also begin to develop the notion of permanency. They have a new appreciation of the consequences of physical impairment. Children with congenital limb deformities or amputations will begin, with new meaning, to talk about how their limbs will never be normal; children with diabetes will begin to talk about having to take medication for "the rest of my life." They begin to understand that what they are experiencing is different from what other children go through and are able to say "it isn't fair."

Along with the concept of permanence comes an increased understanding of the concept of death. Children at this age, if given the opportunity, may ask if they are dying. Those who do not ask may, nevertheless, welcome the reassurance that they are not dying.

At the same time that latency-age children appear to be making rapid intellectual progress, they may continue to harbor old fears and anxieties. Under stress children and adults alike often regress to fears and fantasies from earlier development levels. Short term psychiatric intervention is often effective in allaying underlying anxiety and facilitating good psychological adjustment.

Preadolescence and Adolescence

Preadolescent and adolescent youngsters are more able to understand the causative factors, consequences, and sequelae of illness. Although in some ways their understanding approaches that of adults, they have little in their past to reassure them, and there is a readily evoked sense that they are being cheated of all that life had promised them. The case of an 18-year-old girl illustrates this poignantly.

Janna was referred to a psychiatrist when the diagnosis was made of a malignant brain tumor. Janna and her family were distraught. Janna recounted that her doctor had told her that she did not have long to live and that she was "in shock." Life seemed so unfair. One week earlier she had felt that she had all the time in the world to do the things she had always wanted — now she had nothing. She had spent her whole life preparing for a future she would never have.

The instinctual drives of adolescence are powerful. Even youngsters faced with their own mortality strive for increased independence, identification with their peer group, and sexual identity (Tisza, 1976). Problems of modesty and ownership of body make illness and hospitalization extremely difficult for the adolescent patient (Schowalter, 1977). At no other time do patients seem so sensitive to anything which interferes with their physical attractiveness and prowess or which singles them out from their peers. Despite the knowledge that her death was imminent, Janna used her free time to practice walking with a cane so that she could go to the movies without the use of a wheelchair and without calling attention to herself.

Although illness and hospitalization pose psychological problems for children of all ages, the consequences seem to be worse for younger children and for those whose confinement is prolonged. Levy (1945), in an oft-quoted study of the psychiatric sequelae of surgical procedures, found that 20 percent of the children in his sample, ranging in age from under 12 months to 15 years, developed significant psychological symptoms after surgery. More striking, while about one third of the overall group was three years of age or less, two thirds of those with emotional sequelae were three years or less. Aside from a higher frequency of severe responses, children in this age group experienced a greater intensity of response than did children in the older group. Douglas (1975), in a longitudinal study of children admitted to the hospital, found an increased risk of behavioral disturbance with a single admission of more than a week's duration or with repeated admissions before the age of five (in particular, between the ages of six months and four years). Quinton and Rutter (1976) confirmed Douglas' findings. Both groups found disorders to be more prevalent among children who came from stressful environments.

Given preschool children's incomplete emotional development, under-developed cognitive capacities, tenuous reality testing, and minimal actual knowledge of their bodies, it is understandable that they are at particular risk (Pearson, 1941). Many young children who are scheduled for surgery are poorly prepared for what they are about to undergo. For most, it represents their first separation from their parents. Many are not given adequate information about where they are going or what will happen. They enter a strange environment, full of hustle and bustle, undergo physical examination and blood drawing, forgo breakfast, and then are whisked off to surgery by strangers.

Menninger's (1934) compelling description of the child's experience of surgery underscores the terror.

> Certainly there is nothing in the practice of medicine so barbarous and fraught with psychological danger as the prevalent custom of taking a child into a strange white room, surrounding him with white-garbed strangers, exhibiting queer paraphernalia and glittering knives, and at the height of his consternation, pressing an ether cone over his face and telling him to breath deeply. The anxiety stimulated by such horrors is probably never surpassed in the child's subsequent life.

In many instances, psychological symptoms following surgery remit in a relatively short time. In other cases, symptoms may not become manifest until long after the operation, at which time it may be difficult to make the connection between the behavior and the procedure. Analytic cases of adults who have undergone surgery as children underscore the far-reaching emotional consequences.

Lipton (1962) presents the analytic case of a young woman who had a great interest in ballet. She performed publicly with extreme gratification. She enjoyed the illumination by bright lights and the sense that she was the object of continuous attention, although she could scarcely see or hear her audience. It was of utmost importance for her to keep their attention and evoke a response — applause precisely geared to the end of her performance. Late in her analysis she vividly recalled her tonsillectomy. She recounted lying on a table under bright lights, hearing a dim mumble of voices, and glimpsing unfamiliar forms. She recalled the feeling of being watched and the fear of an unknown danger. Her hope was to ward off the danger by lying perfectly still. By the perfection of her behavior/performance, she hoped to evoke *no* response from the shadowy threatening figures around her. This case material suggests that consequences of surgery in childhood may have a profound organizing effect on ego development without necessarily being adaptive or maladaptive.

EFFECT OF THE CHILD'S PERSONALITY AND LIFE EXPERIENCE

Having reviewed the influence of a child's age and development on the reactions to hospitalization and surgery, let us consider some individual differences that may affect the outcome. Of these, one of the most important is the child's premorbid personality and ability to handle anxiety. Some children are easygoing and good-natured. They seem to roll with the punches. Others seem from birth to be sensitive to even the most mildly unpleasant stimulus. In general, the more psychologically healthy the child, the better equipped he is to weather the storm of hospitalization and surgery.

Another potent factor molding children's response to illness, hospitalization, and surgery is their previous life experiences. Children who have recently experienced a significant change such as the birth of a sibling need time to master the event before facing another trauma. They may benefit from the postponement of elective surgery until their emotional reactions have become stabilized. Children who have suffered unusual trauma, such as a separation from their parents or the death of a relative, are at risk for heightened anxiety and psychological complications and may need psychiatric intervention before their admission.

RELATIONSHIP WITH THE PARENTS

Another critical factor influencing children's response to hospitalization and surgery is their premorbid relationship with their parents. It is generally agreed that a good parent-child relationship correlates strongly with a good outcome after hospitalization (Pearson, 1941; Prugh et al., 1952; Douglas, 1975). Psychological disturbance following illness seems to occur most frequently in children whose parents have a negative attitude toward them or are most psychologically disturbed (Pearson, 1941; Prugh, Staub, Sands, Kirschbaum & Lenihan, 1953; Gibson, 1965).

Whatever the premorbid relationship, hospitalization and surgery themselves inevitably affect the parent-child relationship. Some parents are unable to visit frequently because of distance or because they are overwhelmed by their own feelings and cannot tolerate visiting a sick child. Most parents, however, respond to illness by hovering over the sick child, giving undivided attention, and responding to the child's every whim. This is confusing and frightening to some children but is gratifying to others.

For children in large families, this may be the first time they have been in the sole possession of their parent's attention and care. These children may find it difficult, upon recovery, to give up emotional gains (Freud, 1952). Thus, sickness may become a source of secondary gain, and the child may express his need for attention through somatic complaints.

To further compound the problem of psychologic recovery, some parents are unable to give up seeing their child in a sick role. Green and Solnit (1964) described "the vulnerable child syndrome" in which parents, unable to work through their child's brush with death, continued to see the now-recovered child as still at risk, highly vulnerable to serious illness or accidents. These children, fretted over excessively by their anxious parents, later exhibit separation difficulties, hypochondriasis, and school underachievement. There is often a disturbed relationship between the formerly ill child and siblings, who are resentful of the parental treatment of the "sick" child as "special."

MEASURES TO REDUCE THE PSYCHOLOGICAL CONSEQUENCES OF HOSPITALIZATION

Although many of the factors which contribute to the child's reaction to hospitalization and surgery are well understood, the physician has little control over them at the time the child is admitted to the hospital. The eve of a major surgical procedure is hardly the time to begin altering a child's personality or relationship with parents and siblings. However, some comprehension of these crucial areas may help the staff to understand, anticipate, and deal with the psychological consequences.

Whenever children are admitted into a hospital, it is important to learn from them what they understand about their admission and to clarify any misperceptions. With children, as with adults, preparation for a traumatic experience helps to reduce the ensuing anxiety. Many parents, however, are so anxiety ridden and guilty that they cannot bring themselves to adequately prepare their child for what he is to undergo. Pediatricians and child psychiatrists are familiar with "pragmatic lies" (Coleman, 1950) that parents tell children to lure them to the hospital.

When Kara was five she underwent a tonsillectomy. Her mother, anxious about the surgery, did not want to frighten the patient by telling her she was to have an operation. On the morning of the surgery, Kara was told she was going with her mother to visit an aunt at her house. As she approached the hospital, Kara noted with surprise that this was not where her aunt lived. Within minutes she was at the door of the clinic, being placed on a cot by two burly attendants, who whisked her off to day surgery. For many years subsequent to her operation, she was unable to trust either her mother or doctors.

In contrast to parents whose anxiety prevents them from giving any preparation, some parents are driven to grossly overdo the preparation in an exaggerated way. Jessner et al. (1952) cites the case of one mother who, beginning six weeks prior to surgery, played out each detail of the hospitalization process, going so far as to lay the child on the kitchen table and to place an ammonia-soaked rag over her face in order to simulate anesthesia. Such examples leave little wonder that the child often becomes a bewildered and terrified patient.

For parents whose relationships with their children are poor, preparation often takes on the negative aspect of the relationship. Children in this situation are particularly prone to see hospitalization as punishment.

Good preparation need not be complicated. Like adults, children need to know the facts. They need to have this information imparted to them in a simple and truthful way, meaningful to them at their age and level of development. They need to get a general idea of what the hospital will be like and what will be done to them. They need to be told that these things will be done to make them healthy and they need to be reassured, realistically, that their parents will not abandon them. Even children as young as three or four can gain some understanding of illness from simple preparation. Children younger than this benefit most from reassurance that they will not be abandoned.

Timing of the preparation is another issue. For young children, two to three days is generally regarded as adequate, while for older children, one to three weeks is preferred, with longer preparation time reserved for the older end of the spectrum. It is recommended that detailed preparatory information about procedures be given after the child is admitted, shortly before the procedure is to be undertaken. Children need enough time to call into action some coping mechanisms, yet not so much time as to become overwhelmed by fear (Freud, 1952). The goal of preparation is to develop not only an intellectual understanding of what will happen, but an "inner preparedness" (Jessner et al., 1952).

Parents' attitudes toward the upcoming hospitalization and surgery will inevitably color the child's reaction to the event. Mothers who are adequately prepared themselves are, in general, better able to adjust to the hospital stay than mothers who are poorly prepared (Skipper & Leonard, 1968). Confidence in the physician, possession of adequate information about the hospitalization and surgery, and (once the child is in the hospital) a supportive relationship with the primary nurse all contribute to the parents' sense of comfort and to their ability to provide comforting preparation and support for the child.

In addition to direct verbal preparation from doctor or parent, the child may benefit from other methods of preparation. Home preparation booklets, to be read by the child and parent together, particularly booklets addressing the child's specific operation, seem to improve adjustment (Wolfer & Vistintainer, 1979).

There is evidence that modeling reduces anxiety. Children viewing a film of other children calmly receiving anesthesia or preparing for and recovering from similar surgery will be less frightened when anticipating their own anesthesia and surgery (Melamed & Siegel, 1975). Modeling may be particularly useful for younger children (three to four) who may respond better to preparation done visually than verbally (Ferguson, 1979). Likewise, brief puppet therapy has also been found to be useful in reducing preprocedural anxiety (Cassell, 1965).

The success of preparation depends to a large extent on the child. As has been seen with adults, those children do best who are not highly defensive and who are able to tolerate moderate anxiety sufficiently to allow fantasy material into their thoughts and play, so that they may engage in the "work of worrying" (Burstein & Meichenbaum, 1979).

SYMBOLIC MEANING OF SURGICAL PROCEDURES

Whatever the site of disease, anesthesia and the actual operation stir considerable anxiety. While younger children seem most concerned about needles, older children focus on the threat of being put to sleep, which they may equate with death, especially those children who have the experience of a pet "put to sleep" by the veterinarian. For some, narcosis is interpreted as a murderous or sexual attack. While some children fear the loss of control when they are asleep, others feel reassured that the sleep will protect them from pain.

Fear of narcosis can often be reduced by a preoperative visit by the anesthesiologist. Such a meeting gives the anesthesiologist an opportunity to develop a relationship with the child, understand his apprehension, provide information, clarify distortions, and offer reassurance regarding the fact that the child *will* wake up after the surgery but will not awaken during the procedure and will *not* feel pain. Aside from diminishing emotional trauma, this method of preparation has been found to be of value in producing quieter induction as well as necessitating less anesthetic agent (Jackson, 1951).

Operations themselves may have many meanings. Most often, they are associated in the child's mind with mutilation or castration. Sometimes they are associated with punishment. For the healthy child undergoing an elective procedure, fantasy-based concerns are heightened; for a child in pain, concerns are often more concrete, and the surgery may be seen as a relief to suffering. Frequently operations are associated with giving birth. At other times, they are associated with sexual change. Sometimes they are confused with surgeries other family members have had. For young children in a large family, certain procedures, like tonsillectomies, which older siblings have undergone, become viewed as rites of passage.

Specific preparation for the surgery itself may allay some anxiety. It is important for the surgeon to develop a trusting relationship with the parents and the child. A private conversation with the parents, in which they can express concerns and receive realistic reassurance from the surgeon, can do much to ease the preoperative anxiety of parents, who in turn can be supportive to the child. Even with the young child, the surgeon must try to establish a rapport and offer reassurance in simple terms.

SYMBOLIC MEANING OF SPECIFIC DISEASES

Certain illnesses or injuries arouse specific anxieties based both on reality and on fantasy. Much research has been done on children undergoing tonsillectomy. Although the procedure is a fairly benign one, usually performed electively in relatively healthy children with ample time for preparation, there is evidence that psychological upset is disproportionate to the realistic significance of the surgery. Jessner et al. (1952) and Blom (1958), who studied children at a time when tonsillectomy was performed to cure conditions ranging from sore throats to enuresis, found that some children, like their parents, saw their tonsillectomies as a panacea. Their tonsils were viewed as "bad stuff" that had to come out. The procedure had a moral connotation, and surgery was viewed almost as an exorcism. For other children, tonsils had a more specific symbolic meaning; tonsils were equated with testicles, eyes, and teeth, and surgery was generally seen as representative of castration and mutilation.

Genital surgery, too, is well-known to evoke castration anxiety for patients at all levels of development. Blotsky and Grossman (1978), in a comparison of children who underwent otolaryngological surgery with those who underwent genital surgery, found that despite psychological theories describing displacement of anxiety and fear of bodily mutilation of non-genital organs, the child cathects the genitals in a "special" way and that surgical manipulation of genitals has particular meaning in contradistinction to manipulation of other bodily parts.

All surgeries can have far-reaching symbolism beyond the direct effect on the patient. Congenital anomalies raise parental concern regarding guilt and responsibility. Mothers are well-known to focus on specific facts and fantasies of their pregnancy and delivery. When the patient is a male with a genital anomaly, there is particular focus on the father's maleness and on the son's sexuality. Siblings are also affected. Moore (1975), in his report of a young boy who had undergone genital surgery, demonstrated the anxiety-producing effect such surgery can have on male siblings.

Cardiac surgery evokes fear of death. Older children as well as adults see the "uninterrupted beat of the heart as evidence of life and its cessation as meaning death" (Meyer, Blacher & Brown, 1961). The heart also has symbolic meaning as the seat of emotion. Young children for whom such abstract conceptualization is incomplete generally tolerate uncomplicated cardiac surgery without the acute postopererative psychological disturbance common to adult patients.

In addition to heart and genitals, Blom (1958) and Langford (1948) noted brains and eyes to be invested with unconscious significance and found surgery on these organs to be particularly traumatic. McRae (1955) noted that surgical procedures involving the ends of the alimentary canal or genitals may have a great effect on personality formation because of the symbolism associated with these areas and their significance in terms of child development.

The reaction to amputation, like that to cardiac surgery, varies with age. Amputations performed before the age of two are thought to be accepted into the body image (Earle, 1979). After that time, they serve as a threat to both body integrity and body image. Children, like adults, grieve the lost limb and are concerned about what has been done with it. Like adults, they experience a phantom limb; however, in the case of young people, the phantom limb is not usually painful. A child's adjustment to amputation depends to a great extent on the parents' acceptance of both the child and his body. Children with supportive parents and previous good body image adapt best to their loss. Case reports by Plank and Horwood (1961) and Healy and Hansen (1977) give evidence that a carefully constructed prosthesis doll is helpful to the child in preparing for the surgery itself and treatment procedures.

SYMBOLIC MEANING OF POSTOPERATIVE TREATMENTS

Postsurgical treatments bring their own anxieties and responses. Dietary restrictions may make a child feel deprived and unworthy. Injections may be seen as physical assaults, and painful dressing changes may seem more like punishment than caring treatment.

Restrictions of movement have been studied extensively. Children are generally active, even when they are sick. Immobilization requires the inhibition of their major form of discharge and anxiety. Several authors have reported on the connection between the restricted limb and other parts of the body. Levy (1945) noted the association between restraint of limbs and the occurrence of ticlike movements elsewhere. Bergman (1945), although she did not corroborate this finding, noted an increase in autoerotic stimulation pointing out that many authors see tics as masturbatory equivalents. In addition, she reported that the restraint of one limb may spread in the form of inhibitions to other parts of the body with resultant inhibition of verbal expression and restriction of mental development.

For the most part, children on orthopedic floors conform to the limitations placed on them. It has been noted, however, that during the restriction and while the restraints are being lifted, there is a general and sometimes longlasting increase in aggression. In addition, while the deprivations necessitated by treatment are tolerated, any chance deprivations or disappointments are reacted to with extreme aggression and distress (Bergman, 1945). The usual expression of this aggression is through restlessness, irritability, and the use of foul language (Freud, 1952).

PSYCHOLOGICAL MANIFESTATIONS AFTER DISCHARGE FROM HOSPITAL

Most children experience some psychological reactions during hospitalization. The dominant reaction is anxiety. In young children, anxiety focusses on separation, with its attendant feelings of loneliness and desertion; in older children the concern focuses on the operation and anesthesia. Even a good adjustment to hospitalization can deteriorate under the stress of continued separation, procedures, and restrictions.

After their discharge from the hospital, in the safe setting of their home, most children display mild, transitory reactions. For the most part, these last for only a week or two and consist of increased demanding behavior, irritability, depression, and occasional nightmares or other sleep disturbances (Levy, 1945; Jessner et al., 1952; Prugh et al., 1953; Blom, 1958). These have been considered as manifestations of the integration of the experience (Levy, 1945; Jessner et al., 1952). However, as many as 20 percent of children may experience more severe or persistent reactions (Levy, 1945; Jessner et al., 1952). It has been suggested that an even higher rate of severe or persistent reaction might be found if the follow-up period were longer (Jessner et al., 1952). Persistent symptoms include severe anxiety (including nightmares of being held down or chased), speech changes (especially in children who have undergone tonsillectomy), tics or mannerisms (especially involving the site of surgery), fear of hospitals, white coats, bodily harm and death, depression, regressive behavior, and (especially in boys) aggressiveness (Levy, 1945; Jessner et al., 1952; Prugh,1953; Blom, 1958). Severe reactions have been reported to be more common in younger rather than older children and in those with premorbid neurotic tendencies, poor relationships with parents, or previous experience of psychological trauma. The best adjusted children are older, able to transfer positive relationships with their parents to staff,and enjoy the camaraderie of other children (Jessner et al., 1952; Blom, 1958). Children master trauma best when they can verbalize and express anxiety in their play and can work through their trauma in fantasy by turning passive into active. The outcome is also better for children in whom reality-based concerns dominate over fantasy-based concerns. These children seem less likely to have later reactivation of anxiety than those children who suppress the experience, adapting superficially but betraying anxiety in their dreams (Jessner et al., 1952).

Evidence suggests that adequate preparation, liberalized hospital programs including flexible visiting hours, assignment of a primary nurse, and the presence of consistent staff at stressful times during the hospitalization all contribute to reduced fearfulness (Vistintainer & Wolfer, 1975) and a better posthospital outcome (Prugh, Staub, Sands, Kirschbaum, & Lenihan, 1953).

There is speculation by some that for a small percentage of children the experience of surgery can actually have a beneficial effect. While most feel that the traumatic aspects far outweigh any positive aspects, Jessner et al. (1952), Blom (1958), and Vernon, Schalman, and Foley (1966) point out that the child can grow through learning and that he can master anxiety and withstand environmental changes. The child may also derive comfort from learning that reality may not be as frightening as fantasy. For some children such surgery as tonsillectomy may signify a right of passage or a gain in prestige within the family or among peers. For others, it might allow an improvement in a condition that previously impaired adaptation.

Most clinical studies do not cover a sufficient postsurgical interval to examine delayed reactions or later reactivation of symptomatology. Reports in psychoanalytic literature, such as that decribed by Lipton (1962), demonstrate at the very least a subtle, long-range effect of early operations on the ego, extending into areas far removed from the original trauma.

CONCLUSIONS

Illness, hospitalization, and surgery are important events in the psychological lives of children. The child's response to surgery depends on age and developmental level, personality, life experience, relationship with parents, and, to a certain extent, on the treatments involved. Anesthesia and surgery each evoke specific concerns based on reality factors and fantasy. The dominant manifestation in the hospitalized child is anxiety. Certain children are at higher risk than others of a marked reaction but in all instances, adequate preparation and appropriate reassurance are helpful.

Most children experience some psychological distress as a result of hospitalization and surgery. At least 20 percent of children demonstrate serious or more persistent reactions, often lasting long after hospitalization. Much more difficult to assess is the role that hospitalization and surgery may have in the development of character. Analysts treating adults give cogent evidence of the profound, lifelong effect that such experiences may have on ego organization. Deutsch (1942) summarized this aptly when she noted that "operations performed in childhood leave indelible traces on the psychic life of the individual."

REFERENCES

Bergman, T. (1945). Observation of children's reactions to motor restraint. *Nervous Child, 4,* 318–328.

Beverly, B. I. (1936). Effect of illness on emotional development. *Journal of Pediatrics*, *8*, 533–543.

Blom, G. E. (1958). The reactions of hospitalized children to illness. *Pediatrics, 22*, 598–600.

Blotsky, M. J., & Grossman, I. (1978). Psychological implications of childhood genitourinary surgery: An empirical study. *Journal of the American Academy of Child Psychiatry, 17* (3) 488–497.

Burstein, S., & Meichenbaum, D. (1979). The work of worrying in children undergoing surgery. *Journal of Abnormal Child Psychology, 7*, 121–132.

Cassell, S. (1965). Effect of brief puppet therapy upon the emotional responses of children undergoing cardiac catheterization. *Journal of Consulting Psychology, 29;* 1–8.

Coleman, L. L. (1950). The psychological implications of tonsillectomy. *New York State Journal of Medicine, 50*, 1225–1228.

Deutsch, H. (1942). Some psychoanalytic observations on surgery. *Psychosomatic Medicine, 4*, 105–115.

Douglas, J. W. B. (1975). Early hospital admissions and later disturbances of behavior and learning. *Developmental Medicine and Child Neurology, 17*, 456–480.

Earle, E. M. (1979). The psychological effects of mutilating surgery in children and adolescents. *Psychoanalytic Study of the Child, 34*, 527–546.

Fergusen, B. F. (1979). Preparing young children for hospitalization: A comparison of two methods. *Pediatrics, 64*, (5), 656–664.

Freud, A. (1952). The role of bodily illness in the mental life of children. *Psychoanalytic Study of the Child, 7*, 69–81.

Gibson, R. (1965). Trauma in early infancy and later personality development. *Psychosomatic Medicine, 27*, 229–237.

Greene, M., & Solnit, A. (1964). Reactions to the threatened loss of a child: A vulnerable child syndrome. *Pediatrics, 58*, 58–66

Healy, M. H., & Hansen, H. (1977). Psychiatric management of limb amputation in a preschool child: The illusion of "like me—not me." *Journal of the American Academy of Child Psychiatry, 16*, (4), 684–692.

Jackson, E. B. (1942). Treatment of the young child in the hospital. *American Journal of Orthopsychiatry, 12*, 56–63.

Jackson, K. (1951). Psychologic preparation as a method of reducing the emotional trauma of anesthesia in children. *Anesthesiology, 12*, 293–300.

Jessner, L., Blom, G. E., & Waldfogel, S. (1952). Emotional implications of tonsillectomy and adenoidectomy on children. *Psychoanalytic Study of the Child, 7*, 126–169.

Jessner, L., & Kaplan, S. (1949). Reactions of children to tonsillectomy and adenoidectomy, In Senn (Ed.). *Problems of Infancy and Childhood: Transactions of the Third Conference* (pp. 97–118). New York: Josiah Macy, Jr. Foundation.

Langford, W. S. (1948). Physical illness and convalescence: Their meaning to the child. *Journal of Pediatrics, 33,* 242–250.

Levy, D. M. (1945). Psychic trauma of operations in children. *American Journal of Diseases of Children, 69,* 7–25.

Lipton, S. D. (1962). On the psychology of chilhood tonsillectomy. *Journal of the American Academy of Child Psychiatry, 17,* 363–417.

McRae, R. I. (1955). The impact of childhood surgery on personality. *Journal of the American Osteopathic Association, 54* (8), 497–500.

Melamed, B. C., & Siegel, L. J. (1975). Reduction of anxiety in children facing hospitalization and surgery by use of filmed modelling. *Journal of Consulting Clinical Psychology, 43,* 511–521.

Menninger, K. A. (1934). Polysurgery and polysurgical addiction. *Psychoanalytic Quarterly, 3,* 173–199.

Meyer, B. C., Blacher, R. S., & Brown, I. (1961). A clinical study of psychiatric and psychological aspects of mitral surgery. *Psychosomatic Medicine, 23,* 194–218.

Miller, M. L. (1951). The traumatic effect of surgical operations in childhood on the integrative functions of the ego. *Psychoanalytic Quarterly, 20,* 77–92.

Moore, W. T. (1975). The impact of surgery on boys. *Psychoanalytic Study of the Child, 30,* 529–548.

Pearson, G. H. J. (1941). Effect of operative procedures on the emotional life of the child. *American Journal of Diseases of Children, 62,* 716–729.

Plank, E. N., & Horwood, C. (1961). Leg amputation in a four-year old. *Psychoanalytic Study of the Child, 16,* 405–422.

Prugh, D. G., Staub, E. M., Sands, H. H., Kirschbaum, R. M., & Lenihan, E. A. (1953). A study of the emotional reactions of children and families to hospitalization and illness. *American Journal of Orthopsychiatry, 23,* 70–106.

Quinton, D., & Rutter, M. (1976). Early hospital admissions and later disturbances of behavior: An attempted replication of Douglas' findings. *Developmental Medicine and Child Neurology, 18,* 447–459.

Robertson, J. (1958). *Young Children in Hospital.* New York: Basic Books.

Schowalter, J. E. (1977). Psychological reactions to physical illness and hospitalization in adolescence. *Journal of the American Academy of Child Psychiatry, 16,* 500–516.

Skipper, J. K., & Leonard, L. C. (1968). Children, stress, and hospitalization: A field experiment. *Journal of Health and Social Behavior, 9,* 275–287.

Tisza, V. B. (1976). Psychological implication of renal transplant. *Journal of the American Academy of Child Psychiatry, 15,* 709.

Vernon, D., Schulman, J. L., & Foley, J. M. (1966). Changes in children's behavior after hospitalization. *American Journal of Diseases of Children, 3,* 581–593.

Vistintainer, M. A., & Wolfer, J. A. (1975). Psychological preparation for surgical pediatric patients: The effect on children's and parents' stress responses and adjustment. *Pediatrics, 56,* 187–202.

Wolfer, J. A., & Vistintainer, M. A. (1979). Prehospital psychological preparation or tonsillectomy patients: Effects on children's and parents' adjustment. *Pediatrics, 64*, 646–655.

— *CHAPTER THREE* ————————————

Heart Surgery:
The Patient's Experience:

RICHARD S. BLACHER, M.D.

Because of the special role the heart plays in our psychic life, heart surgery, though common, is never commonplace. While in the United States alone well over 200,000 major cardiac procedures are carried out each year, the emotional impact this surgery has on the patient makes it enormously different from surgery on any other part of the body. For the patient, heart surgery is unique in several ways. First, it is often elective and yet experienced as life endangering. Second, no other organ is so connected with the idea of life and death. As one patient said, "I know that other organs are vital but the heart is the *most* vital organ in the body." Another patient summed it up well by saying, "The heart, after all, is the heart of the body." Here the metaphor was more important than the reality.

Our culture equates the beating of the heart with living, and although *we* have come to accept a flat EEG as the indication of death, to the patient it is the absence of a heartbeat that serves as this marker. Prior to any other surgery, patients worry that during surgery their hearts will stop and they will be dead. Cardiac patients have a further problem: they must accept the fact that during the operation their hearts will be stopped (many patients have seen the procedure on television and thus know what to anticipate, even if they have not been told about this aspect by their doctors). They then must worry about "the moment of truth" when the surgeon restarts the heart. This has implications which will be discussed later.

Aside from its centrality in life and death, throughout history the heart has been considered a special organ, inspiring awe. It is intimately associated with love, other emotions, and even intellect. Thus, a painting of Jesus showing his heart is a religious symbol and numerous churches "of the sacred heart" attest to this. It would be hard to consider a church labeled "sacred pancreas," or "liver," or even "brain" without seeming ludicrous.

Undoubtedly, primitive man recognized that the heart ceased beating with death. In addition, he was aware that he could experience his heartbeat at times of both exertion and great emotion — anger, fear, or sexual passion. Thus, the connection was made with both life and death and emotional states.

The idea that the heart is considered by the primitive as the source of courage (derived from the latin *cor*) is reflected in cannibals eating the heart of fearless enemies. Certain North African tribesmen avoid eating fowl heart lest they become overly timid. The North American Indian has also associated the heart with courage.

Eating the heart obviously was quite common in the days of early Egypt, since the *Book of the Dead*, as quoted in Boylan (1969), proscribes this practice. Ancient Egyptians felt that the heart represented life and death and thought that it gained a few grams of weight each year until the fiftieth birthday, when it began to lose the same amount of weight until death. In order to enter paradise, one had to be judged by the God Osiris, who weighed the heart in a scale against truth, represented by a feather.

Aristotle considered the heart as a source of blood and innate body heat and felt that it must also be the origin of sensation and thought. The brain was thought of as a cold gland preventing the body from being overheated by the heart (Boylan, 1969). During the Middle Ages, numbers of kings and prominent clergymen had their hearts buried in one church and their bodies in another and several prominent people, such as Edward I of England and Robert the Bruce of Scotland attempted to have their hearts buried in Jerusalem. This practice of separate heart burial has continued to modern days. Byron's and Shelley's hearts are both preserved. The explorer David Livingston had his body sent from Africa to Westminster Abbey but his heart was buried in Africa. As recently as 1937, the heart of a Canadian monk and miracle worker, Brother Andre, was removed and placed in a special urn that is touched by the faithful in his church in Montreal (Boylan, 1969).

Today informed people recognize the importance of the brain in thought, emotional reactions, and personality, but this "silent organ" still does not have for the average person the dramatic qualities of the heart. Nowhere is this reflected more than in the languages of the world. Expressions such as light-hearted and heavy-hearted indicate emotional states. Having one's heart in one's mouth indicates fear; a change of heart suggests more than a change of mind. Even intellectual functions are involved when one recalls something by heart. The hyphenated use of the heart is not restricted to English but is seen in all languages, although some ancient Persian poetry will substitute heart-liver in place of the usual words involving heart. To have heart means to be both brave and compassionate as opposed to heartless and chicken-hearted. While there may be references to other organs in our language, such as "guts," these references are infrequent (Meyer, Blacher, & Brown, 1961).

Patients facing cardiac surgery carry with them all the burden of the past meanings of the heart in their culture, although the background of illness and expectation of treatment may be different from one cardiac condition to the next. For example, patients with rheumatic heart disease may often come to operation with a history of knowing for 20 years that someday they might need surgery. On the other hand, some patients are admitted with very brief histories of angina pectoris with a work-up revealing the necessity for immediate surgery, such as in those patients with significant left main artery disease. These patients have very little time to prepare themselves for the operation. Obviously, between the time of the catheterization and the scheduling of the surgery a varying degree of time may elapse, sometimes because of the wishes of the patient who may want to spend time getting his affairs in order, and sometimes because of the exigencies of a busy hospital operating schedule. The decision as to whether an operation should be done or not is itself one fraught with a great deal of ambivalence. If patients are told that surgery cannot be performed they accept this as a death warrant. On the other hand, if they are accepted for surgery then they must undergo what they experience as a life-threatening situation.

Different patients have different waiting times which might be considered by them as ideal. An informal survey of people reveals a range from one day to several months as the time they would like to delay a procedure on themselves. However, very few patients can dictate the terms, as did an eminent cardiac surgeon a number of years ago (Starr, 1976).

This surgeon called his catheterization team in on a Sunday morning because he noticed some symptoms. Following catheterization he decided that he needed surgery, but when the team suggested scheduling him for the near future, he was able to veto the suggestion and call for an *immediate* procedure. Of course, one must consider that his requesting catheterization indicated that he was already somewhat prepared for a coronary bypass graft.

If the patient must wait a month or two, he lives in a state of suspended animation, with a certain degree of anxiety that bubbles up occasionally. However, despite a previously high level of anxiety, on the day before surgery one often sees a dramatic decline of tension. The patient will attribute this to the careful and detailed explanations given by the surgical team, but this must be understood as a rationalization because such explanations to the layperson might be expected to increase anxiety rather than diminish it. What we see is a massive denial taking place. Since the greater the perceived danger, the greater the need for denial, one would expect such patients to show more denial than patients about to undergo other general surgical procedures. Indeed this is so.

In a study of pre- and postoperative patients (Meyer, Brown, & Levine, 1955), patients who were on a general surgical floor were given House-Tree-Person tests before and after surgery. The psychiatric consultant described the subjects as mildly anxious preoperatively, and in general, as calm postoperatively. Both pre- and postoperative tests were given and the psychologist who read the paired tests blind was able to tell which were the preoperative forms with 100 percent accuracy. He described the patients showing severe anxiety, even approaching psychosis preoperatively, and a tendency to return to normal after the surgery was over. The same psychologist reading paired pre- and postoperative House-Tree-Person tests on a series of cardiac surgery patients was incorrect in 66 percent of the cases (Brown & Blacher, unpublished data). What was characteristic of the preoperative patients was the massive denial. The fact that postoperative patients might be more disturbed should not be surprising in this surgery when the denial is given up *after* the patient survives. It is not uncommon for a person to feel calm while going through what he experiences as a life-endangering situation such as being in a skidding automobile and to respond with the appropriate action to preserve his life. When the danger has passed, however, it is usual for a wave of anxiety to sweep over the participant. That this is not due to a sudden outpouring of catecholamines after a few seconds of danger is evidenced by such experiences that have occupied longer times, even up to an hour.

Another dramatic aspect of cardiac function is the fact that the heart is the only organ that works in an obviously binary fashion; it is either off or it is on, and people will talk about someone being one heartbeat away from death. It is for this reason, as well as that the patient considers heart surgery to be so dangerous, that an almost universal fantasy is that the mortality rate is 50 percent. "You either live or you die," is often stated, and even though patients are told about the true mortality rate, which may be less than 1 percent in an uncomplicated coronary procedure, they nevertheless feel that they have a 50–50 chance. Discussing this anxiety and emphasizing the real knowledge may at times be anxiety-relieving.

Another thought that may upset the patient in anticipation of surgery was summed up by an anxious patient, who was highly educated, had listened carefully to the explanation of the surgeon, and seemed to understand the procedure thoroughly, yet still asked the question, "when they take my heart out and put it on the machine, will they keep it in the same room with my body?"

This fantasy of the heart being taken out of the body is not rare. In a series of patients studied for their understanding of the procedure after a careful explanation given by the surgeon (with a demonstration using a heart model to illustrate valve replacement) 6 of 30 patients had the concept (Blacher, 1971) that the heart or the heart and lungs were removed during the surgery and placed on a machine—the heart/lung machine. Numbers of these patients did not believe that their hearts were opened in order to replace the valve. And it is not uncommon for patients to view the position of their valves as outside of the heart itself; there is usually a transmural migration of the valve from inside the heart into the large vessels. The patient may tolerate having his heart removed, but not having it opened.

The lack of knowledge about the anatomy of the heart is not surprising. While the heart is the most highly cathected organ, its component parts for most laymen are not known, and the physician should not assume that the patient understands a verbal description or a demonstration with a model.

The patient becomes extremely confused when he tries to conceptualize what is going on in his body. For instance, patients with septal defects are often told that they have "a hole in the heart." This conjures up all sorts of pictures, and patients may say "The hole in my heart allows the blood to run into my lungs and then I become short of breath." This confusion of language is common in medicine and especially so in cardiology where the patient is often unduly frightened by cardiological terms that have a different meaning in the vernacular. An expression such as "congestive heart failure" seems to be a terminal diagnosis. "Heart block," while an EKG finding to the physician, is seen by the patient as a literal obstruction of blood going to or coming from the heart (Blacher & Levine, 1976).

An occasional patient worries greatly that when opening the chest, the surgeon will discover the presence of a lung tumor. Naturally this anxiety is most common among cigarette smokers or those who have had family histories of lung cancer.

In my experience, the most common cause by far for severe anxiety preoperatively is the fantasy that during surgery the patient will be dead and his soul will go to heaven to visit lost loved ones. When the surgeon starts the heart again, the patient will then feel in conflict about whether to stay or return to his regular life. Patients who are most vulnerable to this conflict are those who have lost a close member of the family, usually in early years, and who have a geographical view of an afterlife (Blacher, 1983).

In all cultures, death is seen not as the end of life, but rather as an altered state. Freud (1915) stated, "It is indeed impossible to imagine our own death; and whenever we attempt to do so we can perceive that we are still in fact present as spectators . . . in the unconscious every one of us is convinced of his immortality." The concept of immortality is a compromise. People can accept the fact of their own demise but only if they deny annihilation. Thus, Freud speculated, "It was beside the dead body of someone he loved that he invented spirits." Freud's interest brought the idea of an afterlife out of the areas of religion and philosophy and into the field of psychology. There has always been a universal preoccupation with life after death and resurrection which was assigned to myth, religious belief, and symbolism. Some of the most dramatic episodes in the Bible are the raising of Lazarus by Jesus and Jesus' own resurrection.

In recent years, we have encountered a new phenomenon, namely resuscitation after cardiac arrest. Although such episodes are common, everyday occurrences in our hospitals, they are always dramatic episodes. When a newspaper headline reports such an event it usually states "Person dies — is brought back to life by doctors." Since death is commonly equated with the cessation of the heartbeat rather than with a flat EEG, such a concept is not strange and is not restricted to the naive and uneducated. For example, a sophisticated surgeon who could not sleep the night before his own cardiac surgery said to a colleague, "I know that they keep your vital functions going when they use that pump—I have used it myself—but with your heart stopped, you are *really* dead." Thus, for the surgical patient the idea of resurrection after cardiac arrest acquires another dimension. The patient can anticipate and contemplate the procedure rather than having to deal with the sudden massive trauma that the cardiac arrest patient must face. It is as if he is sitting beside his *own* body rather than that of the loved one noted previously (Freud, 1915). In other words, *the cardiac patient deals with the idea of dying as actual rather than as symbolic or metaphorical*. Such a concept may, in vulnerable patients, prevent them from having necessary surgery.

Case 1

A 46-year-old chemist came for psychiatric consultation because of her ambivalence over a suggested coronary bypass. Her severe angina pectoris made her active life torture, and yet she was not able to understand why she felt that she would die during the surgery despite the reassurance from the surgeon that her prognosis was excellent. The patient's mother had died of heart disease when the patient was 10 and she spoke warmly of the very close relationship she, as an only child, had with her mother. She had given up religion in adolescence after a strict Catholic upbringing. The patient spoke of her knowledge of the operation and kept returning to the stopping and starting of the heart. "When the heart stops it is dead. Not you, but your heart." She kept returning to two things—her close relationship with her mother in early life and her concern about the heart stopping. It was suggested that her fear of surgery was due to the fantasy that when her heart was stopped her soul would leave her body, go to heaven, and join her dead mother. When the surgeon restarted her heart she would then be in conflict between staying in heaven with her mother or returning to life. To this rather wild-sounding interpretation she responded with an eager nod and stated, "You hit it on the head." She made clear her relief that she could now talk about this fantasy. Shortly after she felt comfortable enough to sign the operative permit. She underwent surgery and had a quick and uneventful recovery.

Case 2

A 53-year-old businessman was so anxious prior to surgery for a mitral valve replacement that cancellation of the procedure was contemplated. Despite his symptoms, he had avoided the operation for over a year because of his certainty that he would not live. He began talking spontaneously of his father who had died when the patient was 12, and as he spoke of still missing him his eyes filled with tears. He revealed that he had been dreaming of his father for several nights and when a similar interpretation as in the previous case was made, namely that he felt he would go to heaven during surgery and then would not know whether he wanted to stay with his father or rejoin his own close-knit family, he replied, "That's *exactly* what I've been thinking."

Case 3

A very anxious 60-year-old woman was troubled by a dream of her brother, a priest who had died 10 years before of heart disease. He appeared, and in an uncharacteristically angry way stated, "I am very disappointed in you." When asked how she thought surgery was performed, she replied that the upsetting part was that during the procedure she knew that they stopped your heart, "And that is like being dead." When I suggested to her that she was worried since she must feel that during the surgery her soul would go to visit her brother, she nodded eagerly and burst out, "But I don't want to stay there—I want to come back to my husband. I've decided that already." We talked about this and we both agreed that since she felt her brother would be in heaven for eternity he could wait awhile longer for her.

In all of these patients, there was immediate relief of anxiety following my interpretation. The patients made it clear that the fantasy suggested to them was conscious, but obviously not something anyone could feel free to talk about. My statement gave them permission to talk of a matter usually not thought of as in the medical realm.

A useful technique in lowering preoperative anxiety is the statement to the patient that the interviewer will see him the next day in the intensive care unit. This statement, often given casually but with a sense of certainty, frequently elicits an expression of relief from the patient. At this time, patients do not need statistics or qualifying statements; they look for absolute expectations on the part of the interviewer that the patient *will* be there on the morrow. Making such an appointment serves this purpose (Kennedy & Bakst, 1966).

INTRAOPERATIVE PERIOD

As in general surgery, the anesthesiologist in cardiac procedures attempts to give as little anesthetic agent as is consistent with proper anesthesia. For this reason, the cardiac patient may on occasion experience awakening while paralyzed (see Chapter 1). Indeed, the traumatic, neurotic reaction to such an awakening was first described in patients undergoing mitral commissurotomy (Meyer & Blacher, 1961). As decribed in the previous chapter the symptoms consist of (1) repetitive nightmares with difficulty in going back to sleep, (2) generalized irritability and anxiety, (3) a preoccupation with death, and (4) a difficulty on the part of the patients in discussing their symptoms, least they be thought insane. The traumatic factor seems not to be the state of being awake, since patients are able to tolerate procedures under local, spinal, or even hypnotic anesthesia. What seems important is the feeling that something has gone terribly wrong, accompanied by a sense of helplessness to do anything about it on the part of the patient. A statement to the fact that the patient was indeed awake acts as a curative agent. This seems to resolve the question that patients struggle with as to whether they actually could have been awake during the surgery. On the one hand they are certain that they were, yet on the other hand they feel that it would be impossible.

POSTOPERATIVE PERIOD

From the early years of cardiac surgery, it has been noted that the rate of psychosis following these procedures has been extraordinarily high, ranging from 20 percent to near 100 percent (Fox, Rizzo, & Gifford, 1954; Kornfield, Zimberg, & Malm, 1965; Blacher, 1972). Kornfield (1965) noted that when the patients were examined by interview rather than by chart study the rate of psychosis was significantly higher. In an early study (Meyer, Blacher, & Brown, 1961) it was observed that when the patients were closely followed by the psychiatric team, the level of major psychic upheaval was low.

In recent years, it has been evident that the percentage of such psychotic reactions has diminished markedly. The factors involved in this change must certainly include improvements in the techniques surrounding surgery. However, psychic factors are probably also involved. In the early days of heart surgery, with its attendant high mortality, patients were treated by the medical and nursing staffs as if they were fragile pieces of porcelain, almost reverentially. The anxiety of the staff was undoubtedly communicated to patients. This played a part in the psychological difficulties as demonstrated by Lazarus and Hagens (1968), who found the nursing staff at first refusing to talk with the patients because of the nurses' anxiety. When they persuaded the nurses to talk to the patients, the rate of psychosis diminished markedly. We have been struck by the fact that it is not only patients with major psychoses who suffer, but also those in whom the psychic distress is more covert. In a way these patients have the potential for greater difficulty, because they hide the upheaval rather than discuss it with their caretakers. Several patients have been seen to worry for over 10 years that they were dealing with a sword of Damocles, anticipating that the psychosis in the intensive care unit after surgery could be repeated at any time. In none of these patients had the difficulty been picked up by the staff during its occurrence. These covert reactions, in my experience, have also diminished markedly.

After surgery, the patient awakens in the intensive care unit where he is subjected to a number of contrasting sensations. In the first place, he experiences relief at being alive. On the other hand, he is subjected to a series of uncomfortable and painful procedures. With tubes and drains in every natural orifice and in several man-made orifices as well, he is wired up to various monitors, lines, and an assortment of equipment. He is usually intubated and therefore unable to speak. Although his obtunded state offers some protection, as he becomes more aware of things the discomfort of his plight becomes evident.

Although some writers have described an "ICU psychosis" (McKegney, 1966), in my experience the psychic situation seems to depend more on what is done to the patient than on the environment. This was shown in an early intensive care unit that housed patients with myocardial infarction, chest surgery, and cardiac surgery. Although the environment was the same, only the cardiac surgery patients developed psychosis. In a fundamentally regressed state, and feeling very uncomfortable, the patient experiences the ministrations of the nurses as torture. Although the sounds and machinery may seem ordinary to the staff, these sounds are stimulating to the patients, and so rather than sensory monotony the patient is subjected to marked sensory overstimulation. Patients would like to be left alone, but the nurses insist on making them take deep breaths, sitting them up, and ambulating them—all this with a painful sternal incision. To express anger is felt to be dangerous, since the patients would expect some retaliation. Even to *feel* this affect is not safe since regressed patients anticipate that the staff can read their minds. Thus, they feel anger but cannot even experience it let alone express it. Not unusually the emotion is projected and the nurse becomes a persecutor in a paranoid system. "I don't want to kill you; you want to kill me," is the patients' theme. This delusion, then, explains why the nurses are hurting them.

Interestingly, the patient does not usually express such a situation openly, but one can easily recognize this state from the suspicious look on the patient's face. Even intubated patients will demonstrate this condition with their eyes and when the examiner questions them directly they will confirm the fact that they feel that the nurses are trying to kill them. Rarely does the physician become a persecutor.

It is possible to ward off this reaction in most cases if the nurses are willing to accept the way the patients perceive them and give the patients permission to feel angry. This is relieving to the patient who will then rarely express negative feelings in an offensive way to the staff. Statements such as "This is an unpleasant treatment and nobody likes it. We expect that the natural human reaction to being hurt is to feel irritable," or "You don't have to like this treatment; you just have to take it," when expressed by an understanding nursing staff can ward off this paranoid reaction almost completely. Even when it does occur, such statements may help somewhat in relieving the situation. Although no control study has been done we are struck by the fact that the absence of paranoia in this cardiac intensive care unit contrasts with the high frequency of such reactions in other surgical ICUs.

Some patients are afraid of moving in the intensive care unit for fear that they will break their sutures—not so much in the periphery as in the heart. These patients respond well to reassurance. This fear of the heart being damaged by movement occurs even in patients who are convinced that their hearts have not been touched during the operation.

ORGANIC REACTIONS

Not surprisingly, the immediate postoperative situation is often marked by some confusion, disorientation, and a mild delirium. For a number of reasons, the patient's cerebrum may be at risk during the operation. About 25 percent of the patients admitted for coronary artery bypass graft have some subtle but demonstrative cognitive dysfunction to start with. This is demonstrable by careful neuropsychological testing (Willner & Rabiner, 1982) or even by a brief mental status testing using serial subtraction and a reciting of the names of the presidents in reverse order. In addition, the heart–lung machine may not provide an absolutely physiological profusion of the brain during the procedure. Such factors as pH, perfusion rates, and pressures are all factors which may play a part in the temporary postoperative brain syndrome.

Strikingly, it is extremely rare for patients in a delirium following heart surgery to tamper with their medical equipment, except for endotracheal tubes. Unlike gallbladder patients who may pull out their T-tubes and catheters, cardiac patients leave such equipment alone, suggesting that even in such a state, the delirious patient's wish to survive remains intact. Such organic impairment may affect the patient in different ways. It may protect him from the anxieties and pains of the intensive care treatment. On the other hand, it may lower his tolerance for dealing with the anxieties attendant on his situation and may make him *more* vulnerable in this way to psychic upheavals.

Perhaps more difficult for the patient than the overt delirium, which can be discussed, is the more subtle cognitive dysfunction that the patient does not reveal to the staff. These difficulties may worry a patient terribly. The preoperative use of cognitive testing can then be used postoperatively to demonstrate the difficulties encountered by the patient. For instance, a patient who could do the subtractions very quickly before surgery might have an enormous difficulty afterward. An example would be a professor of history who explained her inability to name the president of the United States due to the fact that she had not read the newspaper recently. In our experience and that of others (Savageau, Jenkins, and Fratos 1982), this postoperative difficulty is almost always reversible, and patients can be honestly reassured that while their minds are currently not working correctly, they can expect their thinking to return soon to normal.

Patients with previous major cognitive difficulties may be confused for a number of weeks. While it is certainly useful to have a neurological evaluation of such patients, it is usual for them gradually, and sometimes suddenly, to make advances in their cognitive functioning to their *status quo ante*.

DEPRESSION

A common postoperative complication, following heart surgery, is depression. To the alert observer, the diagnosis may be obvious, with a depressed affect, psychomotor retardation, and withdrawal. Some medical attendants, however, may look on these manifestations as a sluggishness due to a major surgical procedure. It is important to make the diagnosis, however, because the difficulty in mobilizing the patient, his lack of appetite, and lack of motion, all may contribute to the development of postoperative complications, such as pneumonia, poor wound healing, and thrombophlebitis. Thus these depressions can be considered medical emergencies.

It was shown (Blacher, 1978; Blacher & Cleveland, 1979) that almost all such patients who develop depression soon after surgery share many similarities. The depression usually starts at a point when the major drains and wires are removed and the patients have a sense that they will survive. Although these patients will tell the examiner preoperatively that they had every expectation of surviving, they reveal after the surgery that they did not think that they would live through the operation, and so the depression, following the unexpected survival, has a paradoxical quality. Before coronary artery surgery was performed, postoperative depressions were rare and all the patients we saw shared a common history, that of the loss of a close member of the family to what the patient felt to be a minor illness or procedure. For example, patients would have siblings who died in childhood following an appendectomy, or a parent who had died young with what had seemed to be a minor complication of diabetes.

With the advent of coronary artery surgery we have begun to see many cases of depression. Our patients' family histories are replete with coronary disease and at times the patient may be the only survivor among a large group of siblings. Almost all of the patients have led fairly normal psychological lives before surgery and have not been previously depressed. Following the surgery, the patients are preoccupied with thoughts of their deceased family members, but mention this only if asked.

Niederland (1968) called attention to a common condition seen in concentration camp survivors who suffered "a chronic state of anxious, bland depression." He labeled this condition "Survivor Syndrome" and talked of the underlying dynamics of regression to archaic oral incorporative levels. These patients suffered because they had survived while others had died. They felt consumed by the guilt that their living had depended on the others' dying. Cardiac surgery patients illustrate another form of what can be called survivor guilt. It is unlike that of concentration camp victims, yet it has certain similarities. The regression is not as great, and oedipal and sibling rivalry issues seem to predominate in the coronary artery surgery cases. Unlike the victims of persecution, postoperative patients have short-lived, easily resolved symptoms. None have needed psychiatric hospitalization.

Both Niederland's patients and the postoperative patients deal with issues of death, one group in a terrifying, chronically malignant setting; the other in a terrifying but brief situation in which the environment is designed to help and rescue rather than persecute. Both feel guilty, in part because of what one can call "the quantitative view" of death. This attitude, shared by many in our society, holds that there is a certain number of deaths required by God or nature, and thus if one person dies, another can be spared. During wartime, if a soldier's comrade was killed in a foxhole that they shared, the survivor would commonly become depressed. An exploration would reveal the theme of "if someone *had* to die, I am glad it was he and not I." This was clearly tantamount to feeling "I am glad *he* died," and an enormous amount of guilt would be engendered, and thus the depression.

For the soldier, a buddy is like a sibling and the buddy's death reawakens earlier death wishes toward an ambivalently viewed loved one. The earlier wish can be transformed into one of wanting a choice. "I wish he would die" becomes "If one of us *had* to die, better he than I." Thus, fate rather than the wish became the lethal agent. This is seen in the surgical patient as well, and the death wishes that were felt to culminate in death for parent or sibling are now revived in the situation of danger to the patient's own life. The choice of who lives and who dies is renewed. In both situations, despite the displacement of the wish, the unconscious wish dominates and guilt and depression result (Blacher, 1978).

A striking difference between postoperative patients and the concentration camp victims is that patients are guilty in response only to old ambivalent wishes rather than to any deeds for which the camp survivor suffers remorse. In addition, postoperative patients are dealing with an acute rather than a chronic situation. (Incidentally this allows treatment to be instituted before the neurosis becomes "fixed." Such rapid institution of therapy, in the early stages of neurosis, seems useful in other conditions as well.)

Case 1

A 48-year-old accountant had been cheerful and optimistic before his coronary artery bypass surgery. Three days following the procedure, at the point where he was transferred to the ward from the intensive care unit, he was noted to be depressed and lethargic. When interviewed by the psychiatrist, he revealed how he had not really expected to live through the surgery and then spontaneously began to talk of the death of his older brother who had died two years before, when he too was 48. The brother had been somewhat of an idol and to a certain degree had dominated the patient. After the brother's death, the patient mourned him appropriately and went on with his life. Treatment for the patient consisted of pointing out to him that his depression was paradoxical, since he had not expected to live through surgery, and by suggesting that it was natural to feel like celebrating *his* successful operation, but that celebration for living must be very hard if someone one loves has died of the same condition. However, the examiner pointed out, the brother's death had nothing to do with his living. Within a half hour the patient was noted to be smiling and moving around his room.

The dynamics of such a treatment will be discussed in Chapter 13 but one can certainly see several elements here. First, there is the loaning to the patient of the interviewer's superego with an implied statement that it is perfectly appropriate to be happy. Second, there is an attempt to dissociate the brother's death and the current situation of *his* living. Unconscious dynamics are not explored or interpreted.

Case 2

A 40-year-old account executive was noted to be profoundly depressed after an aortic valve replacement. She had given the interviewer an explanation for her having avoided surgery for several years by telling of various business and family problems that prevented her taking time off for the needed operation. Her symptoms finally became so bad that she had no choice. She was optimistic about the outcome. After the surgery she revealed that she had avoided the surgery for fear of dying and was absolutely amazed when she realized that she was still alive. She found herself preoccupied with thoughts of a younger brother who had died during an appendectomy while he was a college student. The patient was in her mid-twenties at the time and did not learn of the brother's medical condition until she received news of the death. Treatment here was similar to that given to the first patient and within a day the depression had lifted. In this situation, the patient sought further discussions about her relationship with this younger sibling and entered a brief psychotherapy.

While such early losses make patients vulnerable to postoperative depressions, a protective factor is the history of the loved one refusing medical care. Statements such as "My brother never listened to the doctors and refused treatment," or "He was stubborn and brought it on himself," spoken preoperatively will usually indicate that the patient will not suffer a postoperative depression.

OTHER POSTOPERATIVE DEPRESSIONS

It is interesting that one rarely sees a recurrence of mania or depression in the manic-depressive patient after cardiac surgery. Perhaps the painful experience of the hospitalization acts as punishment, warding off any guilty reaction that might trigger the affective condition.

While the survivor depressions usually occur about the third postoperative day, other depressive reactions may be seen later. There is a general tendency in hospitals to explain away depressions as natural reactions to major surgery. Nothing could be further from the truth. There is usually a clear explanation for any such depressive reaction, although, of course, we may not always be able to ascertain it at the time. Just as the preoperative patients who have surgery canceled react to the existential plight of feeling anger but being unable to experience it safely, so do some patients in the postoperative state. Patients who are highly regressed, as in the intensive care unit, react with paranoia, to what they experience as unnecessary torture. Later, when they feel in less danger, they react to such situations with depression. For example, patients with wound complications such as infections or painful sutures may have to stay longer in the hospital or even be forced to return for further care. These patients are invariably depressed. Sharing with the patient the understanding that it is a natural human reaction to feel irritated by the necessity to extend the hospitalization usually results in a rapid diminution in the depressive affect.

SPECIAL PROCEDURES

Pacemaker Implantation

Pacemakers are currently implanted by a cardiologist rather than a surgeon and are no longer considered unusual. From the patient's point of view perhaps the most significant change in pacemakers has been their mode of function, from that of a steady pacing to the newer demand mode that comes into use only when the patient's heart rate falls below a certain level. This change allows patients to feel that the pacemaker assists them rather than "runs them." The feeling of being controlled is intolerable to a number of patients (Blacher & Basch, 1970), who avoid the procedure despite the fact that their frequent episodes of fainting due to a low pulse rate makes life miserable for them. "It is as if I didn't run my own life," said one woman who had managed to control her own as well as the lives of her family members. She never became reconciled to her postoperative status and remained depressed for many years. Twenty-five percent of the patients in a study of psychological reaction to pacemaker implantation, described the pacemaker as a device for pumping blood — in other words, an artificial heart. It was felt that the implantation was a minor procedure to the physician but not to the patient. The pacemaker is unique as a prosthesis in that it does something to the patient rather than being used by the patient, along the lines of artificial hearts.

Intra-Aortic Balloon Pump

The intra-aortic balloon pump (IABP) is a device that assists the heart in pumping blood via an automatically expanding balloon in the aorta. It is coordinated with the heart function by means of electrocardiographic impulses. No systematic study has been made of patients' reactions to this dramatic device, although some interesting responses have been seen wherein patients attribute to the machine some animate qualities. In one case of machine failure the patient remarked, "The machine died and if I did not get myself away from it I would have gone along with it." Often the machine seems to be considered as part of the general equipment.

The balloon pump, like the pacemaker implantation, is considered a minor procedure by the medical staff. In the not-too-distant future, much of cardiac surgery may also be considered minor—to the physician per-haps—but certainly not to the patient. The emotional impact of having one's heart stopped and touched is enormous and must be borne in mind in trying to understand how patients react to such surgery.

REFERENCES

Blacher, R. S. (1971). Open heart surgery–The patient's point of view. *Mount Sinai Journal of Medicine, 38*;(1),74–8.

Blacher, R. S. (1972). The hidden psychosis of open-heart surgery. *Journal of the American Medical Association, 222*;(3), 305–308.

Blacher, R. S. (1978). Paradoxical depression after heart surgery: A form of survivor syndrome. *Psychoanalytic Quarterly, 47*;(2), 267–283.

Blacher, R. S. (1983). Death, resurrection, and rebirth: Observations in cardiac surgery. *Psychoanalytic Quarterly, 52*, 56–72.

Blacher, R. S. & Basch, S. H. (1970). Psychological aspects of pacemaker implantation. *Archives of General Psychiatry, 22*;(4), 319–323.

Blacher, R. S. & Cleveland, R. J. (1979). Heart surgery. *Journal of the American Medical Association, 242*;(22), 2463–2664.

Blacher, R. S. & Levine, H. (1976). The language of the heart. *Journal of the American Medical Association, 236*;(15), 1699.

Brown, F. & Blacher, R. S. Unpublished data.

Boylan, B. R. (1969). *The New Heart*. Philadelphia: Chilton.

Fox, H. M. & Rizzo, N. D. & Gifford, S. (1954). Psychological observations of patients undergoing mitral surgery: A study of stress. *Psychosomatic Medicine, 16*;186.

Freud, S. (1915). Thoughts for the times on war and death. *Standard Edition, (Vol 14)*, London: Hogarth.

Kennedy, J. A. & Bakst, H. (1966). The influence of emotions on the outcome of cardiac surgery: A predictive study. *Bulletin of the New York Academy of Medicine, 42*, 811–845.

Kornfield, D. S., Zimberg, S. & Malm, J. R. (1965). Psychiatric complications of open-heart surgery. *New England Journal of Medicine, 273*, 287–292.

Lazarus, H. R. & Hagens J. H. (1968). Prevention of psychosis following open-heart surgery. *American Journal of Psychiatry, 124*, 1190–1195.

McKegney, F. P. (1966). The intensive care unit syndrome. *Connecticut Medicine 30*, 633–636.

Meyer, B. C. & Blacher, R. S. (1961). A traumatic neurotic reaction induced by succinylcholine chloride. *New York State Journal of Medicine, 61*;(8), 1255–1261.

Meyer, B. C., Blacher, R. S. & Brown, F. (1961). A clinical study of psychiatric and psychological aspects of mitral surgery. *Psychosomatic Medicine, 23*, 194–218.

Meyer, B. C., Brown, F. & Levine, A. (1955). Observations on the house-tree-person drawing test before and after surgery. *Psychosomatic Medicine, 17*, 428.

Niederland, W. G. (1968). Clinical observations on the "survivor syndrome." *International Journal of Psycho-Analysis, 49*, 313–315.

Savageau, J. A., Jenkins, C. D. & Frates, R. W. M. (1982). Neuropsychological dysfunction following elective cardiac operation. *Journal of Thoracic and Cardiovascular Surgery, 84*, 595–600.

Starr, A. (1976). A heart surgeon tells of his own coronary bypass. *Medical World News*, 52.

Willner, A. & Rabiner, C. J. (1982). The psychopathology and cognitive disorder syndrome (PCD) in open-heart surgery patients. In R. Becker, J. Katz, M. J. Polonius & H. Speidel (Eds.), *Psychopathological and Neurological Dysfunctions Following Open-Heart Surgery*, pp. 59–67. Berlin: Springer-Verlag.

CHAPTER FOUR

The Subjective Experience of Brain Surgery: The Mind at Risk

JOSEPH JAFFE, M.D.

We are interested in patients' subjective experience of surgery. Of particular concern are the more subtle and complex meanings of this experience; these meanings could be the basis for therapeutic interventions that might reduce the emotional stress of surgical procedures and facilitate recovery. Specifically, this chapter compares the symbolic significance of brain surgery with that of operations on other organs in order to emphasize its unique aspects.

Surgery is a major life stress. Contemporary research on life stress demonstrates that the identical event (e.g., loss of a job, or divorce) may have widely differing impacts depending on the *significance* of that event for different individuals' psychic economies. It therefore behooves us to understand the special significance of the illness and the surgery for each patient. Such knowledge would enable us to reduce the obvious stress inherent in surgical procedures.

One would imagine the psychiatric interview as an ideal setting for the exploration of such phenomena. This is true, but with some important caveats. Intense levels of terror, anguish, and pain are generally not conducive to subtlety of expression. Intense time pressure is similarly inhospitable to shades of meaning. For this reason, the psychiatric interviews which seem to yield the richest data are preoperative evaluations of patients who are physically relatively *comfortable* and who are facing *elective* surgery. Conversely, the urgent surgical emergency, so beloved by the mass media, replete with wailing sirens and stretchers racing to the operating room, lacks the contemplative quality that is optimum for the exploration of subjective semantic systems. When everyone's hand is forced, the decision structure is simpler; patient and family don't sit around debating the relative merits of different treatment strategies. The very situation dictates the surgical decision, and psychological shock and disbelief render subjective material unavailable.

In contrast, elective surgery involves identical life-threatening illnesses as do the emergency situations, but without the time pressure and therefore with the patient in a more communicative state. In effect, elective surgery is "calamity by appointment." Furthermore, the delay of the operation provides an opportunity for the emergence and elaboration of hopes, fears, value systems, and fantasies, as well as personal and interpersonal conflicts. Finally, *the delay permits the assessment of coping and recuperative powers of both the patient and his or her social network.*

Thus, the clinical material on which this chapter is based, namely *elective brain surgery*, is carefully selected to maximize the possibility of tapping the patients' habitual, longer-range, nonemergency subjectivity. The results might even shed light on the phenomena of nonelective emergency situations where shock and denial make subjective data unavailable.

ELECTIVE BRAIN SURGERY

With the background just described, let us focus on intracranial illness which has potential life-threatening consequences, but where the operation may be postponed for weeks or months. In these situations the patient is often an active participant in the surgical decision, and can investigate, understand, and debate the relative pros and cons of the contemplated intervention. Once there are such options, a "quality-of-life" decision is in progress and it is in these situations that psychiatric consultation can make a significant contribution by working with the patient as well as with the support network.

What is "elective brain surgery?" Conditions that create this context are intracranial aneurysms, arteriovenous malformations, certain brain tumors, seizure disorders, and insufficient cerebral circulation, among others. What they have in common are symptoms that, even if sudden and severe, are not irrevocably incapacitating. The patient may have been through extensive diagnostic evaluations for other suspected conditions before the diagnosis is made of an intracranial lesion. Several clinical examples will make the point clear.

Case 1

A patient has suffered from migraine headaches for years and a variety of medications have only partially relieved the symptoms. Finally, in desperation, a physician recommends a CAT Scan which suggests a very slow growing tumor of the frontal lobe of the brain, most probably benign. Craniotomy is scheduled in two weeks.

Case 2

A previously healthy patient has had a single epileptic seizure. There has been no recurrence on anticonvulsant medication. However, an astute diagnostician detects a "bruit," (a noise over the skull synchronized with the heart beat that can be heard with a stethoscope). An angiogram is performed and reveals an aneurysm on the surface of the brain. Craniotomy is scheduled two weeks hence.

Case 3

A patient has developed mild memory difficulties which interfere with his professional performance. Careful examination of the carotid arteries reveals a 90 percent narrowing, sufficient to compromise cerebral oxygenation. Carotid endarterectomy is scheduled for the next month.

Case 4

A brilliant student sustains a closed head injury in an automobile accident. A personality change ensues, she drops out of college and becomes irresponsible, alcoholic, and sexually promiscuous. An electroencephalogram reveals a discrete spike focus in the nondominant temporal lobe. Temporal lobectomy is contemplated.

What do these cases have in common? One could live with all these diagnoses, or in spite of them. A century ago, prior to the advent of modern neurological surgery, people did just that. But patients are increasingly well informed and are aware of the incredible advances in diagnostic and operative technique. They read the debates in the medical literature, seek second, third, and fourth opinions, and are frequently knowledgeable about statistical outcomes, even the reported outcomes when the appropriate operation is performed by different surgeons. Each of the cases cited has a possible surgical solution but could also be treated more conservatively.

We will discuss the so-called elective situation because it seems closest to analogous quality-of-life decisions that are made in cardiac surgery or renal transplant, namely, major decisions where real, competing options exist, and where each decision has both virtues and drawbacks. A patient may choose to live with the threat of an intracranial bleed ("the time bomb in the head") rather than undergo aneurysm surgery with its attendant risks. Similarly, awareness that prolongation of life by cardiac bypass surgery is still controversial may result in a patient's decision to be managed medically, and other patients may prefer dialysis to the risk of organ rejection after renal transplant. The mystical, primitive, irrational forces evoked by any life-threatening illness are much more approachable, interpretable, and understandable in these elective situations than in the immediately devastating emergencies where everyone's hand is forced. When we approach the surgical patient in this frame of mind, we discover two phenomena. First, there are common threads in all surgical procedures. They consist of fears of violation of body integrity, fears of mutilation, hopes for instant magical cure, and fears of loss of control (e.g., during anesthesia). Second, the psychological variation among operations on different organs is as striking as the similarities.

One of the most interesting differences among surgical procedures concerns the manner in which the offending organ is perceived in conscious awareness. In other words, "How much and in what way is the organ a part of the body image?"

Some organs, such as the eyes, hands, or external genitalia, are prominently represented in the body image because they can be seen and felt. Others, such as the pancreas and spleen, are "silent" and totally absent from this image. Still others are normally out of awareness but are thrust into consciousness the moment there is a malfunction. Examples of the latter are the heart during an arrhythmia, the bronchi during an asthmatic attack, the thyroid gland in Grave's disease, or the duodenum when ulcerated. Perception of fullness of the stomach, experienced as satiety, has been found to vary widely among individuals and may play a role in eating disorders. For example, the perception of stomach contents can be tested experimentally by introducing different volumes of fluid via an indwelling stomach tube. The patient is asked to tell the difference between say, 10 and 20 cc of fluid. Some patients can perceive the difference. Others, who eat to excess, may not be capable of this discrimination so there may be a physiological basis for a failure to experience the fact of "having eaten enough." Some of us may not receive signals of satiety if stomach volume is absent from our body image. In exploring the symbolic aspects of surgery, we must therefore know the degree to which a given organ system is capable of being represented in the body image and the conditions under which this awareness occurs. In this context we shall see that the brain is not a "silent" organ, but that because of certain unique properties, it appears to be so.

THE BODY IMAGE IS IMAGINED

The body image is a psychological experience. As such, *it occurs in the brain.* Perhaps the clearest demonstration of this assertion is the phenomenon of "phantom limb." In this sometimes difficult neurological problem, the experience of an existing limb persists after it has been amputated. Indeed, the absent limb may be subjectively fixed in a specific posture, such as being flexed at the knee, may be subject to intense cramps, or may be agonizingly painful. For many years, surgeons would carefully examine the surface of the stump of the amputated limb for irritative foci, such as neuromas of the severed peripheral nerves, as a cause for such distressing phantoms. But flexion of an imagined joint at the knee is unlikely to be within the coding capacities of peripheral nerves in the absence of a cerebral representation of the leg itself. Without doubt, the most compelling proof of the cerebral representation of the body image was reported by the British neurologist, Sir Henry Head (Schilder, 1950, p.12). His patient had a garden variety of phantom limb following an amputation. But when the patient subsequently suffered a stroke in the opposite half of the brain, the phantom abruptly *disappeared,* indicating that the phantom was not fabricated. The stroke had abolished the cerebral substrate for the imaginary limb. Subsequent research has revealed phantom phenomena after dental extraction, mastectomy, and rhinoplasty. The body image is obviously more resilient than its peripheral origins.

Stimulation of most organs in the body leads to an anatomical *projection* of the "peripheral" event onto a "central" map in the brain. Projection is a geometrical, and more popularly, a photographic concept. The general idea is that some pattern which is *actually* on the film is physically reproduced (mapped onto) in a place where it really *isn't,* that is on the screen. Thus, urinary urgency may be due to a full bladder, the stimuli from which are projected to the brain which is not itself under hydraulic pressure. The resultant brain event is a psychological reality in which the stimulus is accurately referred back to its point of origin. This spatial referral (there can be temporal referrals as in déjà vu experiences) is another projection, this time in conscious experience, of the "real" brain event to the "imagined" physical environment which is, in this case, the body image of the urinary bladder. We can then say, "I have to urinate." The sentence would not be uttered by a person with a severed spinal cord whose bladder is nevertheless capable of reflex emptying in the abscence of projection to the brain. In the intact nervous system, the self must urinate, not the bladder.

In general, the function of most organs that are experienced consciously, such as the hands, eyes, bladder, rectum, urethra, stomach, larynx, and so on is appropriately located. Thus, the most basic diagnostic question still remains, "Where does it hurt?" Spatial localization of the point of stimulation is very precise on the fingertips and more diffuse on the skin of the back, and on the peritoneum, pleura, and meninges. In certain cases, however, the psychological projection of the source of stimulation is very far from the actual locus. As a result, anoxia of the heart muscle may be experienced in the left arm. A kidney stone may be experienced in the testicle. Pressure on a dorsal root of the spinal cord may be experienced in the foot. In these aberrant cases we say that the pain is neuropsychologically "referred" to a site other than that of the offending organ. Here the spatial map of the projected experience is incongruent with the map of pathological stimulation, which makes physical diagnosis such a fascinating detective story.

SUBJECTIVE EXPERIENCE OF THE BRAIN

If the body image is a brain event, one may ask "How does the brain imagine itself?" Proceeding as before, "How is brain stimulation experienced consciously?"

Dahlberg and Jaffe (1977) have said:

> Of all the organs in the body the brain alone is insensitive. Surgery on the brain itself, once the skull has been opened, does not require anesthesia. The patient can be comfortable and fully conscious. It follows that we cannot experience the brain's activity in the place that it occurs, inside the head itself. Rather, the activity of the brain is referred (projected) to the source and destination of its messages.

This is dramatically demonstrated when a neurosurgeon gently stimulates the exposed brain in a search for an epileptic focus. The patient may experience paresthesias, flashes of light, sounds, voices, or complete visual scenes, but these are experienced in the environment or in the body rather than in the head. "Stimulation of certain locations while the patient is speaking causes acceleration or cessation of speech. The patient is aware of these effects but cannot account for them, being unaware of the stimulus" (Dahlberg & Jaffe, 1977). In short we don't experience brain events where they occur but rather in our bodies and in our surroundings. In other words, brain events are completely referred elsewhere and subject as they are to a lifetime store of memories and expectations, they give rise to a variety of perceptual illusions more wondrous than the referred pain of angina pectoris.

For example, "Where is the boundary of the body? Most of us would probably vote for the skin surface, but that isn't the psychological reality. When the dentist anesthetizes one half of our jaw, it feels much larger than the unanesthetized side. A blind man's body extends to the end of his cane. When parking an automobile we feel the curb with the car's front tire. A painter's skill is in the tip of the brush. When we take off a pair of ice skates, there is a soft cushion between the soles of our feet and the ground. These . . . are very real physical experiences. Instruments that serve as extensions of the body enlarge the body image, and others recognize this fact" (Dahlberg & Jaffe, 1977). When patients carry a cane, people tend to give them more space. We locate important events at the interface between our egos and the environment. And our egos are not limited by our skins. This is the work of the brain, itself insensitive, projecting the boundaries of the body image to where the action is.

But our common sense persists in locating brain events at the physical interface between brain and environment, that is, at the effectors and receptors. Can we then understand the old punishment administered to children for speaking profanity, washing their mouths out with soap? Or a music master striking a pupil on the fingers to correct a note played out of tune? Or the expression, "See no evil, hear no evil, speak no evil." Surely, evil must first be seen and heard before it is understood to be evil and therefore, it must be understood before it can be unspoken. Yet, folklore locates all these events in the mouth, fingers, eyes, and ears, all essentially supplementary servants of the brain.

Where is speaking skill located? Common sense places it in the mouth. When groping for a word which we can't remember, it is often said to be "on the tip of the tongue," because that's just the way it feels. Most people won't believe that the problem is in the brain and not in the mouth because it doesn't feel that way. Let's examine several other examples of the everyday experience of trying to locate a complex skill.

When first learning to play the piano, write, type, or knit, one's whole being seems to be engaged in the task. The neck or back may become stiff with tension, and the tongue may stick out. Total concentration and undivided attention are required during the first painful steps of the learning process. But with continued practice, the task becomes easier and eventually, automatic. The movements become so well rehearsed that they require progressively less attention. One can even begin to woolgather or think about what comes next, while the task runs off almost unconsciously, with less and less effort. At this point, we say that we finally have the particular skill "in our fingers" because that's just the way it feels.

Marc Antony implored the Romans to "Lend me your ears!" This metaphor was a request for the undivided attention of the entire brain; attention to a forthcoming verbal message. Yet he would not have been satisfied had his audience merely listened; he also wanted them to comprehend and to be persuaded. Metaphorical language betrays our naive concepts. We "put words into someone's mouth" rather than into someone's brain or mind. Common sense can obviously be misleading.

We must conclude that normal brain stimulation is *never* experienced in the cranium. It is *always* referred to the body or to the extracorporeal environment. And since brain events are consistently mislocalized, the brain is as silent an organ as the pancreas or adrenal gland, but not because its function is not being reported loud and clear in a manner that can be intelligible to its owner. Rather, the brain is a silent organ because its internal events are totally referred elsewhere. This turns out to be a critical distinction between the perceptual basis for symbolism of the brain as opposed to all other organs that are accessible to conscious awareness. The brain perceives its own function as something else, which it calls the outside world or the body image. Yet it is not itself part of that image.

FANTASIES ABOUT THE BRAIN PRIOR TO ELECTIVE SURGERY

It is instructive to ask many people facing potentially traumatic physical situations to discuss their major fears. This technique has a long history. One such attempt was made by a combat psychiatrist in World War II (Kardiner & Spiegel, 1947). Dr. Spiegel asked soldiers going into combat what injury they most feared. Psychoanalytic wisdom at the time predicted that castration anxiety would naturally select the genitals as the most vulnerable fantasied target. He reports that to the contrary, the most feared injury was to the face and eyes. In the same vein, Blacher, psychiatric consultant on a cardiac surgery service, reports that the major fear of patients about to undergo open heart surgery is sudden death (Blacher, 1983).

Blacher (1983) reported:

> Cardiac surgery provides an experiment in nature whereby patients are confronted with what the average person would interpret as dying – namely, a situation in which the heart is stopped before being operated upon. Usually, the patient has an opportunity to anticipate and think about the situation. Unlike people who are dying of a chronic illness, these patients are subjected to what I have called "acute dying."

A similar finding was expected in brain surgery. However, fears of not surviving the operation were almost never mentioned in a series of about 200 precraniotomy patients. Fears of paralysis or sensory defect (especially blindness) that are mentioned in contemporary informed consent procedures were more common, but still not the most frightening. The most salient fear prior to brain surgery is *loss of intellect*, often described as "becoming a vegetable."

The heartbeat can be felt by everyone. But as previously discussed, the functioning of the brain cannot be experienced directly. It is difficult for anyone to imagine that a lesion in the brain can cause paralysis of a foot. This is counterintuitive. Thus, the function of the brain is popularly conceived, by professionals and laypeople alike, as having to do with "the smarts." Childhood memories of the origins of one's personal organ language referring to the brain commonly include, "a brainy kid," "nobody home," "brainless," "nothing upstairs," "empty-headed," "out to lunch," and the old joke, "When God said, 'Will all those who want brains come forth, he came fifth.'" Furthermore, the commonsense definition of death is cessation of the heartbeat. It is paradoxical that the current medical definition of death is "brain death" rather than "heart death," since brain prostheses do not exist. In fact, the brain is popularly conceived of as a noncritical organ of special competence (such as intelligence), which many people can almost live without, sometimes happily. In summary, the major concerns of craniotomy patients tend to involve less existential, perhaps more abstract symbolic systems than in the case of cardiac surgery.

DISCUSSION

Such contrasts between the fears and fantasies of patients facing threats to different organ systems are instructive for the psychiatric consultant who is responsible for crisis intervention on surgical services. We are warned not to resort to pat generalized psychodynamic formulations. The history of psychosomatic medicine has illustrated this need for differentiation of symbolism according to specific organ systems. Although emotional constellations that enter into the choice of a psychosomatic target system is still controversial, the "ulcer" or "coronary prone" personalities are still viable concepts. The task in preoperative consultation is somewhat easier, since the target organ has been chosen already and its personal meaning to the patient can be explored.

Certain methodological problems should also be mentioned. One might ask, "How representative of human symbolism are these selective surgical situations?" An implicit premise underlies the bias of this study. This premise is that the mind becomes more creative as stress is reduced; that necessity is not necessarily the mother of invention. This notion has been expressed in relation to word association tests, in which a person is presented with a stimulus word (S) and instructed to respond (R) with "the first word that comes to mind"; for example, (S) "white" $\rightarrow$ (R) "black", (S) "good" $\rightarrow$ (R) "bad." The *first* word association that comes to mind is less likely to reflect a deeply held belief than an easily available defense (F. Miale, personal communication, 1960). Pressure elicits clichés, whereas psychological inquiry at a relatively more leisurely pace elicits subtlety and differentiation. Let us carry the argument to a ridiculous extreme. One could argue from these premises that the appropriate context for exploring the surgical experience should be normal individuals who are *not* facing the psychological threat of imminent surgery. The counterargument is one that plagues research in experimental social psychology. It is that if the threat really does not matter in some existential way, one cannot trust the results. An example which springs to mind is the research on normal individuals' susceptibility to being persuaded to inflict torture on their colleagues in contrived experimental situations. They do indeed attempt to inflict it, but would they act the same way if they didn't trust the experimenter? Another example derives from experimental research on hypnotic suggestion. When instructed to touch a live rattlesnake, hypnotized experimental subjects attempt to do so. But would they act the same way if they did not trust the hypnotist? These methodological considerations dictate the compromise solution adopted here. Stress experiences should not be hypothetical, and a requisite degree of reality exists in a true clinical situation. But the emergency aspect must be reduced so as to avoid clichéd responses, for which reason the elective surgery situation is preferred to the emergency one.

In this context, we observe that the brain is not symbolized as the organ of life, but rather as the organ of intellect. The power of this idea derives from folklore and from education rather than from direct experience. The brain is a spuriously silent organ whose normal function is experienced as the extracerebral "body image" and the external environment. Given this misleading reporting system, fantasies regarding one's brain must remain highly metaphorical and unrealistic.

REFERENCES

Blacher, R. S. (1983). Death, resurrection and rebirth: Observations in cardiac surgery. *Psychoanalytic Quarterly, 52,* 65.

Dahlberg, C. C., & Jaffe, J. (1977) *Stroke: A Doctor's Personal Story of his Recovery.* New York: Norton.

Kardiner, A., & Spiegel, H. (1947). *War Stress and Neurotic Illness.* New York: Hoeber.

Schilder, P. (1950). *The Image and Appearance of the Human Body.* New York: International Universities Press.

CHAPTER FIVE

Psychological Factors in Lower Limb Amputations

PETER G. WILSON, M.D. and
MARY JANE SCHIRGER-KREBS, R.N.

Amputation is a devastating, anxiety producing event, which has tremendous impact on the individual over time. Whether done quickly in the midst of an automobile accident, or after much time and thought in a diabetic patient, the preoperative phase (short or long) is fraught with fear, sadness, and anger, and quickly leads to a postoperative time, where the limb is gone and phantom phenomena abound. This is followed by a rehabilitation phase of sweat and toil (with a prosthesis) to get back "up" on one's feet. The patient's life is hacked at not only physically, but also emotionally, as he has to stop working and stop living in the world. Instead he lives in a hospital setting where at first everything is done for him; then much is expected of him, which is to begin functioning normally, with a final thrust "out," back to a world with a different shape, literally and figuratively.

CASE STUDIES

Case 1

Larry, an 18-year-old man/boy, working nights, going to school days, living on his own for the first time, is unloading a truck when he is suddenly rammed by a car and left a bleeding wreck on the side of the road . . . later told that an above-knee amputation must be done.

Larry is at the second individuation phase, where the world is opening up; working and living independently are tenuous but palpable. He is unsure how girls will respond to him and is very vulnerable to rejection. He goes off with "the boys" to drink every weekend, and it is important that "they" see him as a man. Suddenly he is truly stricken down, squashed by the car at the dawn of his manhood. A "helpless" patient at the hospital, he is at the mercy of doctors, nurses, and "others," who have control over him. His leg is trussed up in a pulley arrangement and if he watches the changing of the dressing, he will see a mangled mess that is certainly not the leg he knew and loved (or took for granted), but red, mottled skin and muscle, which is given shape by the bandage. And the pain that comes in two packages: the pain that is there always, dull, demanding, draining, telling you that "it is there" and the other pain that comes in waves, building in crescendo, until you want to scream, but "men don't scream."

His family comes from a distance away: father, mother, and brothers. All are concerned, all want to help. But his father has always been stoic and taciturn and must get back to the family farm. Someone must take care of business, money, and ongoing life. So he goes back. Larry's brothers are at school and after a few days they "have" to return to their studies. His mother remains but that relationship is tricky, because she respects him and wants him to have control . . . and he does too, but he also wants to regress and be taken care of and have her make decisions . . . at least part of him does. The surgeon is a strong, masterful, decisive man . . . "Leave it to me. I'll try to save the leg." Larry thinks, "Aha, a wonderful miracle man who can do it. My leg will be fine, whatever that means." Larry being bedridden is mean and irritable, but the nurses are gentle and kind and even bring pain medication quickly, when he asks. It will be a long time before Larry discovers that you don't wait until you are out of your skull with pain (ready to scream), but ask as you feel it building . . . it will cause less wear and tear on you (and the system) and you will need less of the medicine to control the pain (Perry, 1984). Time moves on, the routine is set . . . friends who called earlier no longer call or come. Only his mother remains, and she plainly wants to return home (yet stay at the same time). The surgeon says, "Looks good," "looks okay," "looks, well . . . not so good." When will this end? One way or the other. Anxiety, fears, lousy food and poor appetite, nightmares and poor sleep, how bad is the pain? All these happen inside, while Larry lies helpless on his back and contemplates his leg and the pulley system. He becomes more demanding of his mother and all the nurses. However, a new person shows up—the mental health clinical nurse specialist. She asks Larry how he "feels" and the dam bursts. All the frustration, fury at the driver who caused the accident, the surgeon, his family, and the nurses who have "failed" him, pours out, washing like a tidal wave over this poor innocent woman. Opening up makes Larry feel somewhat better, although the taste of sadness is bitter on his tongue and heart. The nurse comes regularly and Larry looks forward with happiness and dread to her visits. Larry is curious as to what will come out next, but cautious too for he feels that there is so much pain to deal with, and how can one be so angry, even at people he depends on and "who are doing their best?" But Larry sure is angry! The anger feels like a bottomless well, and his anger blindly attacks everyone. Anger at his father's reticence; his mother's siding with his father in arguments; his brothers getting preferential treatment. One must wonder if there is no end to this anger? The answer: yes and no . . . but some of the angry baggage is left behind and some remains.

After several months, Larry is taken to the operating room for a small procedure, to tie up some blood vessels and repair a muscle and wakes up to be told that his leg had to be amputated.

Larry is stunned. After all this time and effort, he cannot believe he has no leg? It's impossible! The surgeon explains that the "necrotic muscle" just collapsed and peeled away from the bone, leaving nothing to work with and because of this an amputation had to be done immediately. Larry feels that he is a failure. He cannot believe that his leg is to be buried. He enters the "zombie period"—nothing tastes right, sleep is horrible, he needs lots of pain medicine, and he is silent with both the surgeon and the therapist. He believes that they have failed and there is nothing to talk about. In Larry's mind the battle is lost. There is no reason to talk about getting out of bed, going to rehabilitation, or getting a prosthesis. However, Larry does rally and begins to move slowly at first and then faster. At first he feels that at least he can move and there are things to do. His family and the hospital staff all become involved in this phase and optimism is high—and then the time comes to "measure for a leg." An "amputee" comes to talk to him, he isn't young and can't really understand. Larry feels that none of the nurses have shrunk away, although he thinks the surgeon has. His surgeon never comes to visit him anymore, occasionally, but not every two days, like he used to. There is a bitter taste in Larry again (sadness) and the edge of a black cloud is always on the horizon.

Larry's thoughts are filled with anger. God damn complications! Areas don't heal right, the "stump" (what a name, sounds like a dead tree), and the not bad looking prosthesis causes irritation. And then the anger spills out to the world. He threatens to leave just when he is getting ready to leave the hospital.

Larry experiences fear. What will happen outside? In the hospital it is safe, the nurses are nice and *everybody* is sick and not whole. Yet on the outside Larry does not know what to expect. His family comes and tells stories of "heroes," who have "done well in spite of adversity and who are nearly as good as before" (e.g., story of Ted Kennedy's son). It is hard enough for him without this added burden. Larry would rather leave in anger than in fear, because to him it's more manly.

He returns to the hospital to tell stories of going traveling with his brother and the "pitiable" looks that people give him. He says that his prosthesis is "pretty good" and looks alright with long pants, although he does walk with a limp. He reports going back to register for school and feeling apprehensive at the time as to how people will look at him. Will he ever be attractive to a woman? Men seem okay to him. It is galling to live at home again with his parents and one brother, money is tight, and he is unsure about the future and his "case" could take years to resolve. Should he go back to school? Everything seems so indefinite. The sadness is less and the fears are less intense. He is grateful for all the help . . . but things did not turn out the way he, the nurses, and the surgeon wanted.

Case 2

Mr. Noel, a 70-year-old, single, retiree with longstanding diabetes, develops an infection of his toes. He is told that his circulation is poor and that he must have a below the knee amputation due to the setting in of gangrene.

He used to work for the United Nations as a translator, have numerous business acquaintances, be good at his job, have a decent income, eat out occasionally, and see himself as an argumentative (but purposeful) and witty bachelor in a cosmopolitan city. He knew he had diabetes, which he took care of with injections, but it wasn't a large disability or annoyance.

Then comes retirement—less money, no close male friends, and only one woman friend. More and more a recluse he walks about the city to occupy his time. An infection of his foot leads to hospitalization when the infection doesn't clear up. A bypass operation is tried, but his foot doesn't heal. A perfectionist, he "does not suffer fools gladly," and so a late lunch tray or a mistake in the menu leads to a battle between him and the staff. He questions the surgical house staff carefully, usually challenges what is going to happen, and puts the staff down as "incompetents." Only the head surgeon is safe from Mr. Noel's sarcastic bullets. Patients are warned, to keep their distance and soon *everyone* is staying away. Physical complications bring out increasing rage, noncompliance with regimens, and finally threats of leaving or possible law suits. The clinical mental health nurse is called in to "help the staff" who want to stay away and have nothing to do with this monster. The staff is concerned that the patient's noncompliance and "hateful behavior" are increasing Mr. Noel's risk of receiving poor care.

The nurse climbs over the verbal and symbolic barricade to see the monster in his lair and finds a very cultured, eccentric and irritable man, who is deeply depressed. Refusing to be driven away, the nurse stays to fight on Mr. Noel's side—getting him physical aides and talking to him about his depression and discouragement. The gangrene spreads and the doctor recommends amputation, which Mr. Noel refuses. However, he does relent and the surgeon performs a below the knee amputation. This reactivates his active war against the staff. Rehabilitation is difficult, because his poor physical shape leaves little room for getting about without a wheelchair. He experiences poor stump healing, which means that prosthesis fitting is slow. By now, Mr. Noel is behaving like a captured tiger occasionally scratching at his captors (staff), but going along with treatment in spite of threats of noncompliance. Returning home is a nightmare. He savages the visiting nurses and physical therapy people who are quick to run away leaving him alone and helpless. The wheelchair is his only means of locomotion and his woman friend is his only visitor. Again the clinical mental health nurse intervenes, and makes for smoother care with explanations to the visiting staff, but Mr. Noel never emerges from his reclusive existence.

DISCUSSION

Psychological factors in lower limb amputees can be looked at in four different ways: (1) factors emerging in specific time periods (i.e., depression before operation, right after operation, etc.), (2) intrapsychic factors, (3) reactions to outside, reality factors, (e.g., loss of job), and (4) reactions that interface with stages of well being, (e.g., pain).

Symbolism of mutilation is frequent in patients who are about to have amputations (Critchley, 1971; Adamson, Hershberg, & Shane, 1976). It emerges in comments and slips that patients make, such as "All I hear are cutting remarks," and in dreams, where grotesque shapes, bloody carnage, and wars dominate. Patients frequently grab onto parts of their body (not necessarily the leg) with fear that "something bad is about to occur." In the immediate postoperative hospital phase, the bloody and destructive dreams continue and only lessen in six to eight weeks, during rehabilitation. There seems to be a connection of mutilation to age, in that conscious comments regarding mutilation are more frequent in adolescents and postadolescents of both sexes. This is not surprising, since turmoil regarding body image and the "coming into being" of the adolescent is a paramount issue. One patient, Larry, liberally spiced his conversation with "mangled and bloody" vocabulary. The further away from the operative procedure (and its physical complications) the fewer the mutilation symbols and dreams.

Not surprisingly, amputation reawakens castration fears in males and nearly every man studied has wondered how he would "do" in the future. Men who have functioned well sexually over time fear that they will be unable to *sustain* erections and adolescents are frequently fearful that they will be unable to *have* erections.

The women studied are concerned about their "attractiveness." Older women in stable relationships question whether men will be revolted by them, see them as "freaks" who are no longer worthy of love, tenderness, and intimacy. Young women often spoke of "being an unattractive cripple, ready for the dust heap," and unable to attract a desirable man. These types of responses are most frequent in the immediate postoperative phase and again when the woman is about to leave the rehabilitation facility and go back home. Total rejection is the expectation of most amputees. "Grotesque," "monstrous," "repulsive," and "yucky" are constantly used; and thoughts of how can anyone want to be with a "disfigured, deformed or malformed" individual?, are constantly in the amputee's mind.

One of the most important factors that molds the amputation experience is pain and how the individual experiences pain. In the preoperative phase, whether the limb has been very painful or not will be a factor in how much the patient wants to be rid of it and how relieved or satisfied he will be postoperatively. The following is an example.

A 56-year-old man had an increasing pain in his lower leg over a four month period before admission to the hospital. The pain started as an occasional twinge, but gradually it became so intense that he could not sleep with his leg flat on a bed. He had to sit in a chair most of the night so that he could sleep and not be constantly awakened by the pain. This man looked forward to the amputation, hoping that it would end the pain and allow him "get a good night's sleep, lying in bed."

In contrast:

A 70-year-old woman had increasing difficulty walking but had no pain in the lower limb that was gradually turning black. She continued to drag herself around the apartment, was able to do most of her chores, and only came into the hospital because the lower limb became infected, causing fever and a disagreeable odor. She was not at all anxious to have the amputation. She felt that she was getting along all right and couldn't understand that this smelly, but nonpainful limb was a danger to her life.

Postoperatively, the amount of stump pain can frequently be connected to the amount of depression or anxiety that the person is experiencing. In well controlled studies, with patients matched for age, sex, and level of amputation, the group having measurable depression and a high level of state anxiety reported more pain than the group without the psychopathology (Sriwatanakul, Kelvie, & Lasagne, 1982).

Phantom pain and phantom phenomena are not psychological phenomena, but do have psychological connections. Many studies (Critchley, 1971; Parkes, 1973; Solomon & Schmidt, 1978; Carlen, Wall, Nadvorna, & Steinbach, 1978) agree that these phenomena occur early postamputation and frequently go away over a period of time. Other studies (Melzack, 1971; Melzack, & Loeser, 1978) suggest that they may last indefinitely. The extent to which phantom sensation continues as phantom pain has been examined by Morgenstern (1970) and Parkes (1973). Both found that with the person who was phantom pain prone there existed: (1) a history of long illness with several surgical operations prior to amputation and persisting pathology afterwards, (2) evidence of neuroticism, particularly a rigid, compulsively self-reliant personality, and (3) an inability to find work for a year. In addition, Morgenstern (1970) found organic symptoms, psychosomatic symptoms, and recurrent depressions in these patients.

There is no way of getting around the loss, the grief, the bereavement a patient feels throughout the pre- and postamputation period. Many studies have examined the psychological reaction to this loss (Dembo, Ladru-Leviton, & Wright, 1952; Kolb, 1952; Parkes, 1976), and others have particularized it as a grief reaction similar to all human experiences of loss (Pfefferbaum and Pasnau, 1976; Parkes, 1975 & 1976; Tourkow, 1974). Parkes (1975), in his retrospective study on the rehabilitation of patients, clearly links the loss and *ability* to grieve to successful rehabilitation. He distinguishes between the reaction of those whose amputation follows a long illness and those who suffer acute war injuries.

Much of this begins in the preoperative phase when the person realizes that a large piece of his real estate, that is, the body will be gone, and it is perfectly appropriate to mourn this loss and to feel that the integrity of a whole has been violated. In the postoperative period, there is frequently a large element of denial and unwillingness to look at the stump. Only when you have to swing over and try to walk with a nonexistent leg, or when the bandages are changed and you happen to look into the area, or a relative comes in and says, "How does it feel to have one foot?" are you faced with the loss and what this loss means. Dembo (1952) and Hughes and White (1946) describe depression as being most marked in the early postoperative weeks. Parkes feels that this period is a frozen period, where the patients allow themselves to feel few emotions. The experiences of Wilson and Krebs, (1983) and Krebs, Wilson, and Cohen, (inpress) shows that this is a tumultuous period, full of feelings of loss.

In many states the law demands that an amputated leg must be given a burial, and therefore, the patient has to sign for this, which makes the situation all the more poignant. The loss becomes concrete; as one patient said, "It was like saying Kaddish for a part of me." Mourning is normal, melancholia or depression is not, although frequently members of the staff say "what can one expect, after all, I would feel the same way." Depression is different, involves other dynamics, that is, loss of self-esteem, and the treatment must indeed be different. Because of the loss, people with amputations are at more risk from depression than those with routine hospitalization and must be watched carefully.

Grieving increases as one leaves rehabilitation or hospital settings (safe havens) and reenters the mainstream of life. Changes always bring anxiety and the grieving is for the "known." Yet our year follow-up of amputees

(Krebs et al., in press) shows little clinical depression and no connection of this dysphoria to the ability to ambulate.

In the immediate postoperative phase, depression may show itself as acting out or noncompliant behavior.

For example:

A 24-year-old man, whose motor-cycle accident had necessitated an amputation, zoomed around the surgical ward in his wheelchair after the operation, putting himself, other patients, and staff in mortal danger from his recklessness.

A 48-year-old diabetic realtor refused to stick to his diabetic diet and would insist on hopping to the bathroom by himself, often landing heavily on his postoperative stump.

A universal preoperative phenomenon is one in which the patient says, "I won't have the operation, I just won't have it and if it's necessary, I would rather die than have this done to me." At first the medical staff thought that this was a serious depressive symptom with strong suicidal overtones. But when it was found that almost all the patients were willing to have the procedure later and tolerated it without major depressive symptomatology, we realised its true meaning. It is a last desperate attempt at controlling a chaotic, out-of-contol situation.

How one handles the amputation is partly due to how one has handled previous crises of life in general and how one has handled one's life, in particular. Successful life experiences, including a history of overcoming difficulties, results in successful coping with loss of limb.

An 80-year-old, highly successful, self-made businessman with a 13-year history of diabetes, lived by the philosophy, "if an obstacle exists, I will fight to overcome it." In spite of his rigid, controlling nature he was likable, intelligent, and sensitive to the needs of others. This was reflected in the numerous telephone calls, greeting cards, and visits he received daily. His devoted wife of 53 years was at his bedside regularly. After retiring at the age of 77 he continued to be active in a number of organizations and traveled with his wife. The threat of an amputation due to an infected toe led to massive anxiety and depression in this man as he experienced a major loss of control over his body and his life. Following a below the knee amputation, however, his stump healed quickly and he was transferred to a rehabilitation facility. Six months after the amputation, he was walking with a prosthesis, without the aid of a cane or walker, and he had resumed his previous activities. This man approached his amputation and rehabilitation as he had other obstacles in his life — he was determined to overcome it. He had also recently resolved the crisis related to retirement by actively involving himself in meaningful religious and social activities. His role in these organizations gave him a purpose to which he could return.

Prugh (1970) divides life into different developmental stages, where different tasks are to be accomplished, well or poorly. Like Erikson (1950), he feels that successful accomplishment of these developmental tasks makes for successful adaptation at that particular stage and ability to move on to other developmental stages. The patient just described had successfully navigated retirement, was dealing effectively with his despair regarding aging, and was willing to share his wisdom and remaining energy with society at large.

Mr. Noel, our 70-year-old patient, had not succeeded at working through this stage of life. Retirement meant cutting off most of his relationships, which had developed through his work or through his epicurean life style. Instead of sharing his considerable wisdom and energy, he withdrew to a reclusive existence, preamputation, with considerable despair.

Larry, at 18, had just begun to free himself from the parental home, was beginning to live on his own, starting to preen and make his way sexually with women, all within the matrix of change, turmoil, and "becoming an adult."

Coping styles as described by Weisman (1978) come into play with amputees. As an example, the person who's always been in control of his life, who's always had to move, who has never depended on anyone, who cannot tolerate dependence very well, will adjust extremely poorly both to being in the hospital and to returning home when it is necessary to learn how to use the prosthesis and accept the need for some help for the rest of his life. This is what Mr. Noel had to deal with and could barely tolerate in the best of times.

On the other hand, the person whose style allows him to depend on and trust others and maybe even encourage this, is much more likely to allow things to be done to him in the hospital, including the operation, and allow himself to be catered to, taken care of, taught how to use the prosthesis and how to utilize the various nursing and rehabilitation routines of the system.

Denial is rampant throughout the time period we are discussing. In the preoperative period, many patients will not deal with the fact that an amputation is coming; when the operative permit has to be signed, the comment may be made, "but my doctor never told me about it." A number of incidents have been witnessed where the surgeon had painfully explained what had to be done and when it was to be done, and the patient still said "I didn't hear any of it." In the immediate postoperative period, denial manifests itself through patients not raising the cover, gleefully reporting phantom phenomena and phantom pain and "truly believing that the leg is still there." Denial breaks down as it becomes necessary to use the nonexistent leg and the surrounding staff and family batter away at the shallow defense.

The tidal wave of aggression and fury that sweeps over the staff usually arrives after the operation when the denial is breaking down. This is the time when the surgeon frequently remains the good guy and the house staff and the nursing staff become the bad guys. After all, how can you be ungrateful and angry at the person who has tried so hard and done so much to keep you intact and who will continue to be responsible in a major way for your care. It is simply unsafe and not "nice." Nevertheless, the staff becomes fair game because "they're not doing their job." The staff experiences a hateful, difficult patient who emerges from the cocoon, scattering buckshot over the geography. It is now that the staff often asks for help or feels that the patient is crazy and must be dealt with. This is actually one of the best times for an intervention.

The increasing anxiety postamputation frequently shows itself in attempts to split the staff. During this time there's constant complaining to the surgeon about nonfeeling nursing staff "who don't even do anything to make this terrible time easier" for the patient. Specific favourite nurses are told that other nurses are perfectly horrid. They are the good angels, in contrast to those evil devils lurking around. This is a regression to the stage of the helpless child in the face of powerful adults whose only defense is to split them apart and in this way divide and conquer. This regression is common and there is constant fear on the part of the patient and staff that it will be interminable. It usually is not.

Symbolism of death is frequent in both the pre- and postoperative stages. It tends to become quiescent in the rehabilitation phase and reappear strongly at the time of going back to a more normal life style, to home and work. There is the obvious connection to depressive symptomatology, but the symbols are also connected to loss of control (e.g., the time of anesthesia). For a 40-year-old man, active in sports, death in a dream was associated with not being able to play basketball again. Watching the game without being "in" it was equated with death.

DEMOGRAPHIC AND OTHER ADDITIONAL FACTORS

We have focused on the psychological aspects of amputation. However, we are aware (Wilson & Krebs, 1983; Krebs et al., 1985) of additional factors significant in the outcome of this surgery. Elements, such as age, extent of amputation (i.e. below or above the knee), complications following surgery, and family and hospital supports, may all influence the results. A chronic condition, especially with pain and many uncomfortable procedures, seems to make amputation more tolerable than an acute situation.

The length of time between decision and surgery may be very important. Some patients need a period of time to adjust and anticipate the procedure. Others cannot tolerate a delay once they realize the necessity for the amputation.

TREATMENT

Mumford and Schlesinger (1982) have shown that psychiatric treatment is useful in surgical patients. This battle has been fought and won. In this chapter we did not detail types of treatment and psychological interventions, except to say that Viederman and Perry's (1980) psychodynamic life narrative, Glick and Kessler's (1980) family model, and our behavioral model (in preparation), all show considerable promise.

SUMMARY

An amputation makes for a very difficult emotional time. Different psychological issues surface along the time continuum from pre- to postoperative stage and finally at rehabilitation time. Some of these patient issues are predictable and by looking for them, expecting them, and addressing them with patients and staff as they occur all concerned will benefit. The patient will have a greater sense of control over his situation and thus will cope with the related stress more effectively. In addition, anticipation of short- and long-term issues, concerns, and problems with patients, allows him time to prepare for those situations, to anticipate problems, and even to rehearse how he might approach the problems in advance. Similarly, by anticipating potential patient problems with the staff and addressing them as they arise, the staff will feel a greater sense of control and can work more effectively with patients confronting the issues rather than getting into power struggles over them.

REFERENCES

Adamson, J. D., Hershberg, D., & Shane, F. (1976). The psychic significance of parts of the body in surgery. In J. G. Howells (Ed.). *Modern Perspectives in Psychiatric Aspects of Surgery*. (pp. 20–45). New York: Brunner/Mazel.

Carlen, P. L., Wall, P. D., Nadvorna, H., & Steinbach, T. (1978). Phantom limb and related phenomena in recent traumatic amputations. *Neurology, 18,* 211–217.

Critchley, M. (1971). Corporeal awareness (Body-image; body scheme). In J. G. Howells (Ed.). *Modern Perspectives in World Psychiatry* (pp. 130–145). New York: Brunner/Mazel.

Dembo, T., Ladieu-Leviton, G., & Wright, B. A. (1952). Acceptance of loss-amputations. In J. F. Garrett (Ed.). *Psychological Aspects of Physical Disabilities* (pp. 81–97). Washington, D.C.: U.S. Government Printing Office.

Erikson, E. N. (1950) *Childhood and Society*, New York: Norton.

Glick, I., & Kessler, D. R. (1980). *Marital and Family Therapy* (2nd ed.). New York: Grune & Stratton.

Hughes, J., & White, W. L. (1946). Emotional reactions and adjustment of amputees to their injury. *U.S. Navy Medical Bulletin*, 157.

Kolb. L. C. (1952). Psychology of amputee: Phantom phenomena, body image, and pain. *Collected Papers*, Mayo Clin, *44:* 586.

Krebs, M. J. S., Wilson, P. G., & Cohen, D. E. I. (in press). Risk factors and coping in individuals with lower limb amputations. *Vascular Surgery*.

Melzack, R. (1971). Phantom limb pain: Implications for treatment of athologic pain. *Anesthesiology, 35* (4), 409–419.

Melzack, R., & Loeser, J. D. (1978). Phantom body pain in paraplegics: Evidence of a central "pattern generating mechanism" for pain. *Pain, 4,* 195–210.

Morgenstern, F. S. (1970). Chronic pain. In O. W. Hill (Ed.). *Modern Trends in Psychosomatic Medicine 2*, (pp. 225–245). London: Butterworth.

Mumford, E., & Schlesinger, H. J. (1982). The effects of psychological intervention on recovery from surgery. *American Journal of Public Health, 72* (2), 141–151.

Parkes, C. M. (1973). Factors determining the persistence of phantom pain in the amputee. *Journal of Psychosomatic Research, 17,* 97–108.

Parkes, C. M. (1975). Psycho-social transitions: Comparison between reactions to loss of a limb and loss of a spouse. *British Journal of Psychiatry, 127,* 204–310.

Parkes, C. M. (1976). The psychological reaction to loss of a limb: The first year after amputation. In J. G. Howells (Ed.). *Modern Perspectives in Psychiatric Aspects of Surgery* (pp. 515–532). New York: Brunner/Mazel.

Perry, S. (1984). Classical management of postoperative pain. *Infections in Surgery, 3* (2), 115–124.

Prugh, D. H. (1970). Dimensions of personality development. In A. Kisley (Ed.), *Crisis in child mental health,* (pp. 298–303). New York: Harper & Row.

Solomon, G. F., & Schmidt, K. M. (1978). A burning issue. Phantom limb pain and psychological preparation of the patient for amputation. *Archives of Surgery, 113,* 185–186.

Sriwatanakul, K., Kelvie, W., & Lasagne, L. (1982). The quantification of pain. *Clinical Pharmacology and Therapeutics, 32,* (2), 143–148.

Tourkow, L. P. (1974). Psychic consequences of loss and replacement of body parts. *Journal of the American Psychoanalytical Association, 22,* (1), 170–181.

Viederman, M., & Perry, S. (1980). Use of a psychodynamic life narrative in the treatment of depression in the physically ill. *General Hospital Psychology, 3,* 177–185.

Weisman, A. D. (1978). Coping with illness. In T. P. Hackett and N. H. Cassem (Eds.), *Massachusetts General Hospital Handbook of General Hospital Psychiatry,* (pp. 264–275). St. Louis: C. V. Mosby.

Wilson, P. G., & Krebs, M. J. S. (1983). Coping with amputation. *Vascular Surgery, 17,* (3), 165–175.

— *CHAPTER SIX* ——————————————

The Psychological Aspects of Breast Surgery

LAURIE A. STEVENS, M.D.

An operation on the breasts is often a highly charged emotional experience, whether it is performed for cosmetic reasons or to treat a malignancy. The breast has always had great personal and intrapsychic significance (Gifford, 1976, p. 103). In addition to the breast being an easily recognized marker of her gender, a woman's breasts also can represent an important component of her femininity. In recent times, there has been an increased emphasis on the breasts, as reflected in advertising, fashion, art, and societal attitudes. Thus, the breasts now take on additional importance to women.

The breasts are associated with the uniquely female role of motherhood and are functionally and symbolically related to both the nurturing aspects of motherhood and deep seated maternal feelings. As a source of sensual and erotic pleasure, breasts are an integral part of female sexuality and as a sexual stimulant to the male, they are an intrinsic feature of sexual attractiveness. In the context of a woman's total personality, the breast is valued as the symbol of her internalized feelings of femininity, motherliness, and sexuality. This important body part helps to create a sense of worthiness and adequacy that underlies self-esteem (Notman, 1978).

The symbolic importance of the breast is a powerful force that is necessary to consider when a woman undergoes surgery to her breasts. Freud regarded the mother's breast as the child's first erotic object. This first object is later generalized into the whole concept of the child's mother. To the conscious, the breast represents femininity, sexuality, and desirability while to the unconscious, it represents mother (Freud, 1940).

Freud regarded body image as being an essential element in the development of the ego. The body image is a highly fluid and variable process and is strongly influenced by the level of ego integration and degree of regression that exists at any given time (Tourkow, 1973). A woman's psychological reaction to surgery on her breasts depends on a myriad of variables—her preexisting feelings about her breasts' size and shape, their significance in the formation of her feelings of femininity, sexuality, and self-esteem, her object relations, intrapsychic conflicts, and reality factors.

In this chapter, the psychological effects of the major types of surgery that are performed on the breasts will be discussed—reduction mammaplasty, augmentation mammaplasty, mastectomy, and breast reconstruction.

REDUCTION MAMMAPLASTY

Reduction mammaplasty is an operation that is performed often for both aesthetic reasons and symptomatic relief. Plastic surgeons who perform this surgery report that this group of patients is the most satisfied with their surgery and seem to be the happiest of all their aesthetic surgery patients in the postoperative period. Most women who seek reduction mammaplasty have breast hypertrophy and suffer from the physical restrictions that accompany their breast size and weight limitations in the ability to participate in sports and to wear a variety of clothing. Furthermore, they are often subjected to people staring at their chests and being teased about their breast size and have sometimes become very shy and self-conscious around men, especially during adolescence. Many report decreased sexual pleasure from their breasts and diminished sensitivity of their nipples to erotic stimulation.

This group of patients usually has very realistic expectations about the surgical results. The most common reaction in the immediate postoperative period is elation and exhilaration with feelings of enhanced self-esteem and general well-being. After the initial period of elation, there often emerges a new set of feelings that may distress the patient. These disturbing feelings include feelings of loss and grief over the loss of a body part, a disturbance of body image characterized by an inability to assimilate the "new breasts" into her body image, transient fears of dissolution (Gifford, 1976), and sexual disturbances.

Body Image Disturbance. Patients may report fears or dreams about their incisions "opening up and allowing the breast tissue to fall out," about their "nipples falling off," or the sensation that "something is missing." Some will feel that their reshaped breasts are not part of their bodies — "just glued on substitutes." Some patients will become very anxious and rather depressed.

Feelings of Loss and Grief. Some patients may experience the grief and mourning reaction described after the acquired loss of a body part or the loss of a loved one. They may feel enormous guilt over having decided to have such an operation.

Sexual Disturbances. The feelings of loss and grief and the changes in body image can interfere with sexual functioning and sexual enjoyment. In the postoperative period, some women experience decreased sensation in their nipples and others have enhanced sensation in their nipples, which may affect their ability to derive sexual pleasure from nipple stimulation.

The patients with the most positive psychological reaction to reduction mammaplasty had, prior to surgery, never fully incorporated their breasts into their body image and rather had experienced them as external objects and an interference in their social and physical functioning. Familiar comments include: "I never really felt like my breasts were part of me or fit with the rest of my figure" and "I have been waiting for a long time to have this operation because my large breasts are such a burden and an encumbrance." The patients who had mixed feelings about their breasts, prior to surgery, have more psychological problems in the postoperative period. They have had both feelings of disgust about their breast size as well as the notion that the breasts somehow served as a buffer that kept the world "at breast's length" and protected them against physical trauma (Goin & Goin, 1981).

Ultimately, the patients undergoing reduction mammaplasty usually have good psychological outcomes. If a negative postoperative reaction occurs, patients usually respond well to support and reassurance. The patients should be informed that a psychological reaction often accompanies this type of surgery and that it takes time for them to achieve comfort with their new breasts' size and shape. It is helpful if the patients have been informed about this period of readjustment before their surgery and they should be encouraged to express such feelings should they occur in the postoperative period.

AUGMENTATION MAMMAPLASTY

Augmentation mammaplasty, like reduction mammaplasty, results in a satisfied patient. Various studies have shown that despite the technical problems and postsurgical complications that accompany this procedure, there is a high level of patient satisfaction and improvement in quality of life in the women who choose to have augmentation mammaplasty. The women who elect to undergo this surgical procedure are a unique group. They are, on the whole, young, married mothers in their forties who are attractive, verbal, and well-dressed. They also have a higher incidence of marital problems and have in some series, a history of higher than normal incidence of major gynecological surgery (Goin & Goin, 1981). Several researchers have described these patients as having a history of unhappy childhood experiences and of disturbed and troubled relationships with their mothers (Druss, 1953).

Gifford (1976) describes a variety of feelings, fantasies, and expectations that are present in women who seek augmentation mammaplasty. These include the idea that pregnancy has depleted their strength and femininity, as represented by the diminution in their postpartum breast size. Pregnancy is often a joyous time in these patients' lives because their breasts become larger as they swell with milk and they experience an enhancement in the self-esteem and feeling of well-being. Their body image during pregnancy is seen as their "true self" or "ideal self" while their body image prior to or after pregnancy is viewed as inadequate. These women experience a profound sense of deprivation and seek restitution through cosmetic surgery to recover their "true self." Gifford (1976) postulates that in these women there exists an antecedent maturational crisis prior to seeking breast augmentation and that the breast surgery is an effort to resolve this conflict, to restore that phase of psychosexual development when they felt loved, feminine, and confident.

Druss (1953) has confirmed Gifford's hypotheses in his in-depth study of six women who underwent augmentation mammaplasty. Motivational factors in these women included a desire to improve their appearance in others' eyes, to be more desirable to their sexual partners, and to repair a deficiency that they feel is present in the size of their breasts when they gaze in the mirror. Women may describe "extreme self-consciousness when trying on clothing in an open dressing room or while making love" with their sexual partners. They may sadly tell how padded brassiers and "falsies" have not been acceptable substitutes for their "flat chests." Druss found a history of difficulties in the relationships of these women with their mothers, characterized by an insufficient identification with the mother and doubts about their femininity and womanliness. He also uncovered a history of depression which he postulates was probably related to problems in their mothering. The desire for breast augmentation is a result of long standing intrapsychic difficulties.

In observing the reaction to surgery, Druss notes that there is an interesting process that unfolds. After the bandages are removed, there is an emotional discharge (i.e., tears) related to the obvious alteration in body image. Then there is a period of self-exploration—visual and tactile—in order to try to integrate the "new breasts" into their body image and to discover their new bodily boundaries. Ultimately, there is a joyful delight with the cosmetic results of their surgery and an enhancement in their feelings of femininity and improvement in their sexual relationships with their partners.

Druss asserts that augmentation mammaplasty patients seek a reunion with their mothers, who had been unavailable or absent earlier in their lives, through a narcissistic identification. Their now full breasts, the symbol of mother, bestow on the patient in their adult life, a new sense of femininity and improvement in their self-esteem that had not been given to them by their own mothers earlier in life. This inadequate mothering had been, unconsciously, symbolized by their "too small" or "insufficient" breasts and had been repaired by a surgical augmentation in their breast size. Druss feels that the regression that the patient experiences while hospitalized, facilitates this reparative process.

In addition to this group of women who have disturbances in their relationships with their mothers, there seems to be a second smaller group of women who have had happy early childhood experiences and satisfactory relationships with their mothers. This group had felt that they have had adequate breast size, prior to their pregnancy; however, the involution that their breasts underwent in the postpartum period has led to subjective distress. These women seek augmentation mammaplasty in order to restore their breasts to their former, prepartum shape and size. They often make statements like: "I just want my body to be returned to the way it was before my pregnancy—I don't care for these shriveled-up breasts." These patients have a high level of satisfaction with their surgical results and a positive psychological recovery because they are returning to a prior positive body image configuration.

Other possible psychological factors that lead a woman to seek augmentation mammaplasty have been offered by Edgerton and McClary (1958), who describe a theory that breast size is experienced as a measure of a woman's father's love and the feelings of inadequacy in breast size as reflective of a woman's guilt about their love and sexual desire for their fathers. There has not been sufficient evidence to either support or refute these hypotheses.

The psychological contraindications to augmentation mammaplasty are similar to the contraindications to other types of cosmetic surgery. These include: (1) the presence of an existing major depression or psychosis, (2) a patient whose primary motivation for surgery is to please others or who is being pressured by others, (3) a patient who presents a sense of urgency or a demand for immediate surgery, (4) a patient who seeks augmentation mammaplasty for the purposes of exhibitionism or sexual exploitation (Goin & Goin, 1981), and (5) a patient who has unrealistic expectations of the effects of successful surgery on her life.

MASTECTOMY

The discovery of breast cancer is a most disturbing event. Most breast lumps are discovered by the patients themselves. The process can begin with an unconscious discovery through a dream, a fantasy, or a sudden "irrational" fear. Discoveries are often made while performing routine behaviors such as bathing or dressing. In response to the discovery, a woman with a breast lump may use denial, and she may not initially be consciously aware of a mass or irregularity in her breast. One woman described a dream that she had prior to the "actual" discovery of her breast lump:

> I had a dream in which I was looking at my decorated Christmas tree and turned around to do something else. I heard a crash and looked back at the tree only to

see that half of the ornaments on one side had fallen from the tree and lay on the floor in small pieces, shattered. After I had this dream, I knew something must be wrong with my body and in two weeks, with a self-examination, I discovered a lump in my breast.

The observation of a pain in the breast, a dimpling of the nipple, or the palpation of an actual breast lump arouses a massive fear response. The patient may then deny the existence of her symptoms and avoid the seeking of medical care. This use of avoidance and denial often leads to a lag time between discovery and report. This time period is often crucial, depending on the aggressivity of the tumor, the nature of recommended treatment modalities, and the prognosis of the illness. Fears that are generated include fears of mutilation, pain, and death as well as fears of dependency and loss—loss of a body part, of work, of family, and of friends.

Prior to biopsy, there is a great deal of stress on the patient. She is trying to make a decision about her body and trying to understand and choose between treatment alternatives at a time when she is most anxious and fearful and her ability to process and integrate information is impaired. In the brief period of time between a positive biopsy and cancer surgery, the patient may experience a wide range of emotions, from anger to depression to despair, with accompanying sleep and appetite disturbances. With the results of a positive biopsy for breast cancer, the alternatives presently available to women include modified radical mastectomy, simple mastectomy, lumpectomy with axillary dissection and radiotherapy, and perhaps, adjunctive chemotherapy depending on the grade and stage of the tumor.

Psychological Response to Mastectomy

There is extensive literature regarding the psychological impact of mastectomy. Studies (Asken, 1975; Jamison, Wellisch, & Pasnau, 1978; Renneker & Cultler, 1952; Roberts, Furnival, & Forrest, 1972) of post-mastectomy patients describe various alterations in:

1. Mood, characterized by a depressive reaction and a lowering of self-esteem
2. Body image, characterized by a diminished sense of wholeness and a sense of asymmetry and body deformity
3. Sexuality, with a diminished feeling of sexual attractiveness and desirability
4. Femininity, with a notion of feeling and being viewed as less feminine

5. Social and occupational functioning, accompanied by feelings of embarrassment and inhibition of activities
6. Fear of recurrence or spread of the cancer and development of cancer in the opposite breast

The process of coming to terms with the loss of a breast is similar to the mourning for the loss of a loved one. This grieving process includes the stages of denial, anger, despair, and hopefully eventual acceptance. Goin and Goin (1981) describe another stage called "pseudoacceptance" in which the woman does not seem to experience the anger–depression phase. Those women use massive denial to protect themselves from their feelings. They deny that the breast loss has had any impact on their self-esteem, body image configuration, functioning, mood, or sexuality. Mourning for the lost breast occurs in patients of all age groups as the symbolic significance of the breast does not change with age.

There are women who are so distressed about the loss of the breast that they never look at their mastectomy scar nor permit their sexual partners to view their scar. There are a large number of women (30–50 per cent) who experience phantom breast sensations, like itching, numbness, and pain, immediately after surgery and sometimes long after surgery. Some investigators report an increased incidence of phantom sensations in their younger patient populations (Jamison et al., 1978; Weinstein, Vetter, & Serensen, 1970).

The factors that determine the nature of a woman's reaction to mastectomy include the significance of her breasts in the creation of her self-esteem, her feelings of femininity and sexuality, her level of satisfaction with her breast size and shape preoperatively, the quality of surrounding supporting figures, and the prognosis of her malignancy. For example, a woman receiving chemotherapy may have many physiological changes associated with the chemotherapy that need to be distinguished from the psychological changes secondary to the mastectomy. While any woman coming to the mastectomy experience brings her own unique set of attitudes about her sexuality, her sexual functioning, and her self-worth, all experience it to some degree as a degenderizing and dehumanizing event (McGrath & Stevens, 1986).

In understanding an individual woman's response to mastectomy, dream material may often be helpful in reflecting the woman's unconscious experience of the cancer.

One thirty-six-year-old woman who was experiencing phantom breast sensations, described a dream in which she had a large black spider fixed to her chest which she could not remove from her body. In her psychotherapy, it became clear that the black spider in the dream represented the cancer that the patient had imagined to be "black on the inside" and she was then able to express her fears about the potential spread of the cancer as well as allow herself to wonder what had happened to her breast that had been removed during her surgery, whether it had been "buried or burned by her doctor" after the pathological examination. The painful phantom breast sensations abated soon after the exploration of this dream.

Another fifty-two-year-old woman had a dream about the positive effects of her chemotherapy: "a large PAC-MAN ate up the nasty intruders that came to rob my house."

Oftentimes, the emotional consequences of mastectomy are all too devastating and lead women to seek a resolution to this emotional upheaval. Therefore, many seek restitution for the lost breast through a reconstructive procedure.

BREAST RECONSTRUCTION

Women who have undergone mastectomy often seek breast reconstruction in order to repair the damage wrought by the mastectomy, the cancer operation. Factors that motivate women after mastectomy to seek reconstruction include the desire: "to be whole again," "to be a woman again," "to diminish self-consciousness," "to enhance my appearance," "to wear what I please," "for my husband," "for my sexual feelings," "because I wish to remarry," "to be rid of the prosthesis," and "to make me feel better." Breast reconstruction can be performed using a variety of surgical techniques —abdominal flaps, latissimus dorsi myocutaneous flaps, with or without prosthesis and prosthesis alone. This choice of the reconstructive procedure should be made by both the surgeon and the patient, tailoring the reconstruction to the body's existing or desired contour.

The decision to have breast reconstruction is a complicated one involving many variables. There are differing viewpoints in the literature about women's expectations of and decision to have breast reconstruction. Goldsmith and Alday (1971) feel that the women who seek reconstruction are having difficulty in accepting and adapting to the loss of the breast, while, in contrast, Asken (1975) supports the view that reconstruction is the only solution to the real disfigurement caused by a mastectomy.

It is of paramount importance that prior to breast reconstruction, there is performed an exploration of the woman's premastectomy feelings about her breasts' size, shape, and her expectations for reconstruction. Women should be shown a variety of photos of women before and after breast reconstruction so that they may carry with them a visual image of what will be occurring in their surgery and to help dispel unrealistic expectations. Some women will utilize reconstruction as a means by which to have the mastopexy or reduction mammaplasty that they have secretly desired for many years. One woman who had not been asked about her preoperative satisfaction with her breasts was very dissatisfied after her breast reconstruction. She had harbored the fantasy that both of her breasts would be larger after the reconstruction and would improve her prior dissatisfaction with her "flat-chested body." If the surgeon had known this information prior to surgery, augmentation mammaplasty for her normal breast could have been entertained as a realistic possibility and a larger prosthesis be placed in her reconstructed breast.

The timing of breast reconstruction has been a controversial topic. Immediate breast reconstruction (simultaneous mastectomy and reconstruction) has become a more available and better accepted procedure. Compared to delayed reconstruction, it seems to offer, for surgically suitable tumors, the possibility of "restoration" of the lost breast and not merely "replacement." Women with immediate reconstruction have, on the whole, less psychological morbidity postoperatively, with fewer reports of depressive symptomatology, sexual dysfunction, feelings of diminished femininity, and impaired body image. They experience the reconstructed breast more as a part of their bodies, than those patients who undergo breast reconstruction as a delayed procedure (Stevens et al., 1984). Some even describe the reconstructed breast as preferable to their remaining healthy breast, because it is "firmer" and "more youthful" — "my adolescent breast."

Delayed breast reconstruction also leads to improvement in mood, sexual functioning, body image, and feelings of femininity but not to the same degree as with immediate breast reconstruction. Patients with delayed reconstruction experience the reconstructed breast as a "replacement" and often do not integrate it well into their body image. However, delayed reconstruction can ameliorate many of the psychological difficulties that women experience after mastectomy. Both immediate and delayed breast reconstruction seem to offer restitution for the loss of the breast by mastectomy.

Every woman deals with the loss of a breast in her own way. She must adjust to the loss of a body part that has great emotional importance in terms of her sexuality and femininity. When a body part is removed, it takes time for the psyche to adapt to the loss. There has been concern in the past that immediate breast reconstruction would somehow alter or impede the process of mourning and psychological adaptation to the loss of the breast. Stevens et al. (1984), in a prospective study of the psychological sequelae of immediate and delayed breast reconstruction, found that immediate breast reconstruction does not appear to alter this process and that the mourning for the breast loss begins in both groups even before surgery with the anticipation of the breast loss.

It is clear that some proportion of the distress that accompanies mastectomy is related to the resulting disfigurement and damage to the self-image. Breast reconstruction appears to meet the psychological requirements for restitution and provision of a restored self-concept. Although preliminary studies suggest that immediate breast reconstruction reduces the negative emotional sequelae of breast loss more effectively than does delayed breast reconstruction, immediate reconstruction will not be suitable for all patients with breast cancer who require mastectomy. Both immediate and delayed breast reconstruction seem to offer restitution for the loss of the breast by mastectomy and aid in a woman's psychological recovery from the painful experience of breast loss.

REFERENCES

Asken, M. J. (1975). Psychoemotional aspects of mastectomy: A review of recent literature. *American Journal of Psychiatry, 132,* 56–59.

Druss, R. G. (1953). Change in body image following augmentation breast surgery. *International Journal of Psychoanalytic Psychotherapy, 2* (2), 248–256.

Edgerton, M. T., & McClary, A. R. (1958). Augmentation mammoplasty: Psychological implications and surgical indications. *Plastic Reconstructive Surgery, 27,* 279–305.

Freud, S. (1940). Outline of psychoanalysis. In *Standard Edition, Vol. 23;* (pp. 144–207). London: Hogarth.

Gifford, S. (1976). Emotional attitudes toward cosmetic breast surgery: Loss and restitution of the "ideal self." In R. M. Goldwyn, (Ed.), *Plastic and Reconstructive Surgery of the Breast* (pp. 103–107). Boston: Little, Brown.

Goin, J., & Goin, M. (1981) *Changing the Body: Psychological Effects of Plastic Surgery.* Baltimore, MD: Williams and Wilkins.

Goldsmith, H. S., & Alday, E. S. (1971). Role of the surgeon in the rehabilitation of the breast cancer patient. *Cancer, 28,* 1672–1675.

Jamison, K. R., Wellisch, D. K., & Pasnau, R. O. (1978). Psychological aspects of mastectomy: I. The woman's perspective. *American Journal of Psychiatry, 135,* 432–436.

McGrath, M. H., & Stevens, L. A. (1986). Psychological aspects of mastectomy and breast reconstruction after mastectomy. In F. P. Heter (Ed.), *Human and Ethical Issues in Surgical Care of Patients with Life-Threatening Disease.* New York: Thomas.

Notman, M. T. (1978). A psychological consideration of mastectomy. In M. T. Notman and C. C. Nadelson (Eds.), *The Woman Patient, Medical and Psychiatric Interfaces. I: Sexual and Reproductive Aspects of Women's Care* (pp. 247–255). New York: Plenum.

Renneker, R., & Cutler, M. (1952). Psychological problems of adjustment to cancer of the breast. *Journal of the American Medical Association, 148,* 833–839.

Roberts, M. M., Furnival, I. G., & Forrest, A. P. M. (1972). The morbidity of mastectomy. *British Journal of Surgery, 59,* 301–302.

Stevens, L. A., McGrath, M. H., Druss, R. G., Kister, S. J., Gump, F. E., & Forde, K. A. (1984). The psychological impact of immediate breast reconstruction for women with early breast cancer. *Plastic and Reconstructive Surgery, 73,* 619–626.

Tourkow, L. D. (1973, May 2). Reporter of the proceedings of discussion group "Psychic consequence of congenital lack and acquired loss of body parts," Spring meeting of the American Psychoanalytic Association, Honolulu, Hawaii.

Weinstein, S., Vetter, R. J., Serensen, E. A. (1970). Phantoms following breast amputation. *Neuropsychologia, 8,* 185–197.

— *CHAPTER SEVEN* ————————————

Emotional Impact of Gynecological Surgery

MALKAH T. NOTMAN, M.D.

Gynecological surgery involves sensitive and symbolically highly charged areas of the body. The genitals and reproductive organs are not only the source of satisfaction of a central drive but are intimately associated with concepts of femininity, self-esteem, and all the many implications of physical intimacy: being able to create children, establish the social unit of the family, and provide a link to immortality. Even when a woman is not sexually or reproductively active, her sexual organs are meaningful in immediate and less manifest ways. This is true even for organs that do not play an active part, such as the uterus of a postmenopausal woman. Thus, illness and treatment in this area are rarely neutral.

As part of training, the physician is taught to strive for objectivity and is expected not to respond to the "ordinary" and usual personal aspects of physical interactions (Fox, 1957; Fox & Lief, 1963). For the physician to be able to treat a patient with a certain amount of distance and apparent impersonality is important in order to perform examinations and treatments appropriately. This permits a focus on the specific problems, analogous to the creation of a "surgical field." It also protects the physician from repetitive, potentially emotionally draining experiences. The physician learns to use relatively neutral language that also protects him or her from vulnerability. Sometimes this depends on euphemisms, such as the term "end stage" renal disease or even talking about a "terminal" patient instead of someone who is dying. Sometimes distancing or objectifying is accomplished by humor. However, this process can extend to the point where the human aspects of the patient's experience are lost, and the impact of someone's having "trouble" with one's most intimate parts may not be addressed at all. Communication can falter; the patient may not feel able to bring up her questions or concerns or explore the effect of a procedure on her sexual functioning or on her life.

Physicians may not realize that their language is obscure or telegraphic or that they have not been direct or explicit. The patient's anxiety may also play a role in her not understanding what is said or integrating its significance, and these factors combine to produce confusion.

There are also obvious sexual implications of genital examinations. The physician, who sees many patients, may not be so conscious of these meanings at a given moment. However, for most adult individuals, undressing before a relative stranger and permitting physical contact is usually done only in a sexual context, and although the patient may fully understand the reality of the medical examination, the sexual overtones can still be present. Thus, presentation of any problems with one's genitals and genital examinations involving intimate contact with another individual has the potential for a highly personal and sexual impact on the patient and also on the physician. This colors the way in which examinations are perceived—which may be with embarrassment, discomfort, anxiety, and even guilt. Similarly, discussions about the genitals and reproductive organs may be sexualized. Although attitudes towards sexuality have changed in recent years, this is still a potentially embarrassing subject.

ILLNESS AS PUNISHMENT

Being ill is sometimes experienced as a punishment or an indication that there is something "wrong" with the person, and perhaps that one deserved the illness. A complex process develops in which an adult who is ill usually regresses and some elements of childlike or magical thinking appear, including the idea that if one has become ill, one must have done something bad, a derivative from early childhood feelings and internalized prohibitions. An illness involving sexual organs is particularly likely to evoke such a response, since most people have some unresolved conflicts or guilt about aspects of their sexuality. Disease can then be thought of as being the result of some sexual wrongdoing or unacceptable thought or fantasy. It is possible to maintain such an idea in the back of one's mind in the fact of clear cognitive awareness to the contrary. Venereal disease was regarded in the past as a punishment for sexuality. Currently, pelvic inflammatory disease, although precipitated by a variety of causes, including complications of intrauterine contraceptive devices, can be perceived by the patient as a sexually transmitted disease and a punishment for sexual misconduct. This idea, that one has become diseased because of one's sexual behavior is deeply rooted and connected with unconscious taboos and guilt about sexuality. The physical examination of the sick part of the body, and the surgical procedures that are offered to cure it can thus become the targets of these ideas and feelings and experienced as punitive. It may be puzzling to the physician for the patient to have what appear to be excessive or extraneous responses to a procedure.

All surgery creates some anxiety. Even when reparative goals are paramount, anxiety about potential mutilation and loss of control and fear of anesthesia are usually present. Surgery on the genitals and the reproductive organs can evoke buried concerns about the intactness of one's genitals and sexuality. Most people can call on their rational minds, their confidence in the physician, and their knowledge of what to expect to help prepare them for the procedure. Nevertheless, the unconscious aspects of old conflicts exert an influence that can cause greater anxiety and concern than might be expected from the actual nature of the surgery to be performed (Janis, 1958). In addition, the particular meaning of the experience is strongly influenced by the individual's stage of life and prior personal experience. Gynecological surgery involving internal organs, such as the uterus, ovaries, or internal genitals, lends itself to many fantasies. This enhances the possibility of distortion and confusion. Even though the external labia and external genitals are visible, for many women examination of their genitals presents a conflict because it is linked to taboos relating to masturbation. In general, women often have a very unclear idea as to the actual appearance of their genitals (Lerner, 1976). Therefore, even if they examined themselves when experiencing symptoms, they may not be clear about the normal appearance. The sense that in some way one may be harmed or mutilated by surgery is thus reinforced by the hidden nature of the problem.

All surgery involves surrendering control at least temporarily. The care of the patient after general surgery does have regressive aspects. Patients are usually treated in such a way that their autonomy over their own bodily functions is given up. Catheters, bedpans, nasal tubes, intravenous medications, and the passivity involved in anesthesia itself mean that the patient has to be tolerant of a level of regression that may create considerable discomfort, particularly for an individual whose adaptation is one which stresses competence and mastery (Zilbach, personal communication, 1983). The recording of urine volumes, of stools, the confrontation with impaired bodily functions may be particularly threatening to someone for whom mastery of these functions in early childhood was associated with some conflict and stress. It may seem like an abandonment of maturity. This infantilizing treatment is accentuated by the passivity required of the surgical patient. When curare-like substances are used in abdominal surgery, patients who recover some partial consciousness during the procedure report terrifying feelings of helplessness.

The dynamic of the relationship between the surgeon and the patient, particularly in the conventional situation in which the surgeon has generally been male and paternalistic, even authoritarian, plays a part in the regressive infantilizing process. The practice of calling the woman patient a "girl" also accentuates this and is devaluating (Notman & Nadelson, 1978).

In further consideration of the emotional impact of gynecological surgery, it is important to take into account the particular procedure and the underlying diagnoses. The particular time in the patient's life cycle also strongly determines her response. Although many of the anxieties and concerns about surgery are not likely to be altered, the psychological state of the patient is vastly different if she is facing a reparative procedure undertaken in order to improve her sexual life or increase her sphincter control and enhance her well-being than it is if she is being treated for a malignancy.

The significance of the organ to the individual needs to be considered. This may vary from patient to patient and may not be entirely predictable by the surgeon on the basis of his or her own values — a common assumption made about a woman's wish for children was that two (or three or four) were "enough" without fully considering the patient's own wishes. The loss of a uterus or ovaries that are "no longer functioning" in the doctor's view may remove a part of herself that seems integral to the self-concept of the patient. (Bunker, 1976; Notman & Nadelson, 1978; Roeske, 1978)

Sometimes reparative surgery appears to the patient to be a magical way to change oneself. This can be based on unrealistic expectations of a procedure, and in fantasy the surgeon is regarded as a potentially omnipotent magician. Disappointment and anger at the surgeon if these expectations are not met can obviously be great (Goldwyn, 1978). Anger may then be focused on some particular aspect of the treatment which the patient feels was not handled well realistically.

If one is confronted with a problem, sometimes the temptation exists to wish it away. Approaching a problem surgically with the aim "to fix it" may permit the patient not to have to think about it in detail. The idea that the surgeon can repair or cure the defective part and restore it to health, and that, therefore, it will be just as if nothing were wrong may be shared by the surgeon, but the narcissistic blow to the patient of having a particular deformity or anxiety about illness usually cannot be totally erased by having it "fixed." This does not mean the patient must be preoccupied with the problem, but some acknowledgment about its role and meaning for her and an opportunity to understand these are usually helpful in truly resolving it.

LIFE CYCLE CONSIDERATIONS

Since childhood disorders of the reproductive organs and their role in development are considerably different than in adulthood, this discussion will be restricted to adolescence and adulthood.

In early adolescence, menarche ushers in the beginning of reproductive life. It is one of the changes that mark the transition into adolescence. The development of secondary sex characteristics, the changes in body shape, size of the genitals, development of pubic hair, and onset of menses are part of the process of becoming a woman. Although there are many negative feelings about menstruating, for most girls there is also a positive organizing effect on body image (Kestenberg, 1961). It defines the vaginal opening, helps establish normal feminine functioning, and serves as an initiation into womanhood.

Abnormalities that result in delayed or absent menses affect the girl's sense of femininity and gender identity. Those girls who do not begin to menstruate at the time their peers do usually feel some concern and eagerness to menstruate even though the periods themselves can be experienced as a nuisance. Some disorders that are undetected until puberty become manifest when menses do not occur. A minor problem such as an imperforate hymen can be treated easily. Major developmental problems such as uterine or vaginal agenesis and genetic and metabolic disorders are not so easy to repair. Procedures performed in this phase of adolescence may be felt as welcome and helpful. However, there is also the possibility that the need for surgery is perceived as a confirmation of abnormality. In adolescence the rapidity of changes in the body and the necessity to integrate new shapes and even new organs into one's body image and self-concept relatively rapidly requires considerable adaptation by the young girl. Adolescents who are unsure of their new selves are often concerned about their normality, and look at each change with some anxiety, although it may also be eagerly anticipated. Surgery itself may be experienced as an assault or as a sexual trauma. Even surgery that is not directly on the genitals, but involves problems around the perineum or repair of traumatic injuries can also be experienced this way. Reassurance about normality and full explanations can be very helpful.

The following case describes an adolescent who was ambivalent about a nonsurgical approach to her problem and gave indications of more profound disturbance, which was hard to reach. She eventually chose a surgical treatment; some of the same problems then interfered with compliance and undermined optimal functioning with an apparently excellent surgical result.*

Case 1

Ms. J. presented at a local gynecology clinic when she was 16½ years old requesting birth control, as she and her boyfriend of several months had become "involved sexually." Her history revealed primary amenorrhea. Physical examination showed an attractive female with fully developed sexual characteristics (Tanner's Classification A), indicating the presence of ovarian function. On pelvic examination the patient had normal external genitalia; beyond the hymen, a smooth membrane could be indented almost two centimeters to create a vaginal dimple. Further workup including hormonal and genetic studies, IVP, and diagnostic laparoscopy revealed normal female karyotype and absent uterus and right ovary. The diagnosis of Rokitansky-Küster-Hauser syndrome (vaginal agenesis) was confirmed and the patient was taught the Frank method of vaginal dilatation (applying pressure for a fixed time each day using dilators of gradually increasing size) to create a vagina over an estimated period of 3 to 12 months. After several attempts of the technique at home, the patient decided "this is not for me now." She agreed to return for follow-up when she desired treatment of her condition.

The patient returned on the day prior to her eighteenth birthday requesting surgical creation of a vagina. She had continued to date her original

---

* This case was contributed by Dr. Vivian Halfin.

boyfriend and wanted to have the option for intercourse. Treatment possibilities of continued serial dilatation and surgical vaginoplasty were discussed briefly with the patient. A psychiatric referral was made at that time to assist her with any adjustment difficulties she might have to this procedure.

At the time of her initial psychiatric interview, the patient described her condition as having "no opening and only one ovary." She understood that "I can't have any children" and although she was upset by this, she dismissed her concern noting, "I can always adopt." Since the time of her initial gynecological evaluation she had felt "awkward and abnormal" as well as "angry because this never should have happened to me." The patient was able to function as an average student in high school, yet some truancy had occurred in recent weeks. She had some female acquaintances but spent most of her free time with family members or with her boyfriend of several years. His understanding was that Ms. J had a "woman's problem" which could be corrected.

The patient was the fifth of six children. Two older sisters had menarche at 16 and 15½ years of age, while the patient's younger sister had menarche at age 13. The patient's oldest sister and her boyfriend's sister were both pregnant at the time she came to the clinic. One of the patient's two older brothers had had a "drug problem." Ms. J's parents were in their fifties, with the mother, a homemaker, more actively involved in the children's activities. The patient described her parents as "old-fashioned" and reported that they had been distressed to hear that her pursuit of birth control was what led to the discovery of her congenital defect. The patient had no past psychiatric history nor did any family members.

A mental status examination indicated a very attractive adolescent who looked her stated age but appeared made up to look older. There was no thought disorder or suicidal ideation. However, the patient admitted to considering "taking sleeping pills" once or twice; she never acted on these thoughts and could not describe what had precipitated them. Her mood was sad when talking about her condition, and she showed a full range of affect. She did not readily talk about her thoughts or reactions.

Although the patient and therapist agreed to meet weekly, the patient and/or her mother frequently canceled appointments. The patient also dropped out of her senior year in high school and increased her hours as a part-time clerical worker. She did not discuss the reasons and minimized the importance of her decision, while her mother was very concerned about it. During the first few sessions the patient spoke of the treatment options available to her. A review of the details of each option provided an opportunity for the patient to raise questions about her anatomy and sexuality. The patient also talked about how "abnormal and alone" she had felt since her condition was disclosed.

Six weeks after psychiatric treatment was begun, a joint meeting was held with the patient, her mother, her therapist, and the gynecological surgeons. Both treatment options were discussed in detail, and the recommendation was made by the surgeons for the patient to try the dilatation technique, since she could expect an excellent result while avoiding any potential surgical morbidity. The patient favored surgery, but after several weeks of consideration she agreed to try dilatation "in order to avoid an operation." Biweekly meetings with the gynecology nurse to answer questions and reinforce the patient's active role in her treatment were scheduled in addition to biweekly psychotherapy sessions. Once again multiple cancelations ensued.

Three weeks later when the patient returned, she reported having used the dilators only twice. She noted a tendency to feel apathetic and to procrastinate. Sometimes her predominant feeling became one of frustration and she said, "Why do I have to do this? Nobody else had to do this. They all take it for granted." The patient also reported feeling at a "dead end." Thus, the dilatation technique was experienced as a constant confrontation with her deficit and merely served to intensify her feelings of abnormality. Furthermore, it angered her to have to work on her own to correct or replace what was taken away, as she felt, by "external" circumstances. The patient reiterated a request for surgical vaginoplasty, noting that "once I had something there" she could readily perform the dilatations required to maintain its patency.

The treatment team agreed to surgery and helped the patient to prepare with explanations of the procedure and hospital course. She was expected to remain at bed rest for approximately five days postoperatively in order to maximize the chances of the success of the graft. In her meeting with the therapist, the patient focused briefly on the extent to which she would "ever feel normal." She anticipated her postoperative response saying, "I think I am going to feel as though a big burden has been lifted off me."

Surgical vaginoplasty was performed and an excellent result obtained. During Ms. J's hospitalization, she focused almost exclusively on the concrete details of her course. She was unable to talk about the emotional impact of her surgery. Ironically, as she progressed and her pain lessened, the patient became more vocal in her complaints of pain. Eventually she was able to identify the overwhelming emotional component of her pain and to express her disappointment with the need to continue dilatations and thus be reminded of her deficit.

One week after discharge, when the patient returned for surgical and psychiatric follow-up, she appeared shaken and upset. Although usually talkative, she spoke little. She eventually revealed that her boyfriend had broken up with her several days earlier, leaving her feeling bereft. By the following week, the patient was more composed, having decided "not to get close to him" despite repeated requests on the boyfriend's part for reconciliation. The patient was also having difficulty using her dilators properly, and the importance of this was again stressed by her gynecologist.

After a two-month lapse in her visits, the patient returned saying that she had used the dilators only sporadically; some vaginal narrowing was noted. In her meeting with the therapist, it was apparent that the patient's poor compliance was multidetermined. The anticipated and hoped-for instant normality had not occurred and the daily treatments still served as a reminder of the shameful defect the patient still felt. The unfortunate timing of her boyfriend's breakup seemed to confirm the patient's fears that she would never be totally normal. Finally, the patient's poor compliance was a manifestation of her conflict between wanting to be a fully developed active woman versus wanting to be a child with little or no responsibility. A possible predictor of this response was her reluctance to discuss her feelings about the procedure, and her choosing instead to express her distress by canceling appointments and withdrawing from school.

Follow-up visits were again scheduled, but the patient did not subsequently return for any appointments with her gynecologist, plastic surgeon, or psychiatrist.

The woman who has reached adulthood encounters gynecological surgery at a time when she has already consolidated most of her feminine identity and has derived self-esteem from the appropriate and normal functioning of her body. However, she is just as vulnerable to the depreciating implications of being told that something is the matter with her body and particularly her reproductive organs. Reproductively related problems such as abortion, treatment of infertility, and operative delivery form a large portion of the surgery for young women. For some, surgery is performed in the expectation of curing vague abdominal complaints and can serve to consolidate somatizations.

The increased rate of caesarian sections has created considerable controversy. Ambivalence at the prospect of an operative delivery and distress if it has occurred serves to highlight the emotional response of women to surgery associated with "normal" processes. Although for most, the safety of the baby overrides other considerations, many women have felt that the birth is taken over, and, in a sense, "taken away" from them if they have an operative delivery.

A woman who is considered young in contemporary terms or young in terms of career or marital possibilities, such as one who is in her early or mid-thirties, is nevertheless at an age in which in the past and in other cultures, most women have started childbearing and some have completed it. She thus faces the finiteness of the reproductive span often with anxiety about aging (Notman, 1979). Fertility problems after many years of contraception, endometriosis, and pelvic infections precipitate awareness of the limited reproductive span and arouse considerable anxiety and depression, which is sometimes displaced onto the surgical procedures offered to treat them. The intensity of responses to fertility problems with pervasive impact on self-esteem and on a marriage has been discussed elsewhere (Mazor, 1984).

The woman in midlife who has not had children and may appear to have come to terms with this, may nevertheless have wishes and fantasies that make the appearance of menstrual irregularities and the approaching menopause distressing. The physician needs to appreciate the potential that procedures, even a diagnostic dilatation and curettage have to stir up fantasies and arouse concerns.

The following vignette illustrates this problem:

Case 2

A 45-year-old woman, unmarried and facing the dissolution of a relationship of four years with a man, developed menstrual irregularity. She was depressed that these symptoms heralded menopause and that she seemed not to be heading for a marriage that had appeared to be her last opportunity for childbearing. She consulted a gynecologist who recommended a diagnostic D&C and was reassuring about the probable outcome. At a later preoperative visit when the patient was asked to sign the operative permit, the gynecologist in explaining the wording of the permit joked, "That's so I can do anything I want to you." The patient responded to the light tone, understood it as a joke, and went home, only to awaken with a nightmare in which she thought she might have given permission for a hysterectomy.

For the older woman gynecological problems can accentuate concerns about feminity, sexual functioning, attractiveness, and self-esteem. Muscular weakness, particularly changes in pelvic muscles, have been considered "postmenopausal." Menopause appears not to be directly involved in any of these; rather they appear to be related to earlier childbirth trauma, disease, or aging (Notman, 1979).

In the face of the data linking endometrial cancer and prolonged use of estrogen replacement therapy, many women have become reluctant to trust any recommended regime; many do nevertheless agree to procedures that are advised by respected or feared authority without feeling that they have a full option for information or collaboration. Malignancy increases as a realistic concern and also focuses fears about one's functioning and possible defectiveness.

Surgical treatment for malignancy has often focused on survival. In this context, it may seem frivolous or unimportant to consider sexual concerns, yet preserving sexual function can be extremely important in maintaining self-esteem, obtaining gratification for sexual needs and intimacy, as well as sustaining relationships that are supportive.

As illustrative of these issues two procedures will be discussed in more detail: hysterectomy and abortion.

HYSTERECTOMY

Hysterectomy remains the most commonly performed major operation in the United States (National Center for Health Statistics, 1980; U.S. Bureau of Census, 1982–1983). According to the National Center for Health Statistics, a rate of 5.6 per 1000 females had hysterectomies in 1980. There are major variations in rates in different populations both from country to country and within the United States. Over 92 percent of the 19,000 hysterectomies in three New England states were performed for indications other than malignancy (Barnes, 1981).

The psychological impact of hysterectomy is complex; partly the consequences follow from the cessation of menses, in part from the significance and extent of surgical menopause if bilateral oöphorectomy is performed. Social factors are important, such as the way in which a woman without a uterus is regarded, the significance for the partner of the "damaged woman," and his inability to impregnate her. The symbolic and unconscious meaning of the uterus for an individual woman contributes to the effects, as does the experience of the surgery itself. For some women the procedure ushers in the end of the era of "youth" and the beginning of middle age or old age.

Available roles and options other than childbearing and rearing and the investment of and gratifications for an individual in her childbearing role are important.

Although a hysterectomy can leave minor or no physical scars, the experience of mutilation and sense of damage and anger can be profound. Conscious and unconscious influences need to be differentiated; a woman who consciously fears further pregnancies may experience conscious relief following a hysterectomy. An unconscious wish for more babies can result in postoperative depression. If earlier depressive symptoms have been expressed in somatizations, the removal of the uterus can precipitate more manifest depression, which then appears as posthysterectomy depression. Many earlier studies did not include preoperative assessments, so comparisons were not possible.

The subject of posthysterectomy depression has received considerable attention and been the subject of controversy. Lindeman (1941) noted a syndrome resembling agitated depression following pelvic operations. Richards (1974), in an often quoted study, described "post-hysterectomy syndrome with features that included depressed mood, hot flashes, urinary symptoms, fatigue, headaches, dizziness and insomnia." The incidence of reported depression varies. Some authors have found no difference in emotional disturbances after hysterectomy as compared with other surgery.

Methodological problems complicated much of the earlier research; retrospective studies did not account for the preoperative mental status of the woman, variable diagnoses were taken together with nonstandard criteria for depression, and variable methods were compared. More recent prospective studies indicate that depression is greater pre- than postoperatively in patients undergoing hysterectomy for nonmalignant conditions. Greater than average incidence of psychiatric morbidity in women seeking hysterectomy is reported in a number of studies (Gath & Cooper, 1981; Gath, Cooper, & Day, 1982; Lalinec-Michaud & Engelsmann, 1984; Meikle, 1977; Moore & Tolley, 1976).

Nevertheless, those women who appeared to be at risk for posthysterectomy depression were those who were under 40, without organic pelvic pathology whose presenting symptoms were presumably psychogenic, those whose marital supports had been disrupted, and those with a previous history of depression (Roeske 1978, Lalinec-Michaud & Engelsmann, 1984). This reflects a higher level of disturbance about hysterectomy than other surgery and probably a greater tendency to recommend hysterectomy for a range of complaints in women who manifest some degree of disturbance.

Obviously not all women are distressed following a hysterectomy; some are relieved to find no malignancy, to be relieved of childbearing, and finished with distressing menstrual or premenopausal symptoms.

Lower educational and other sociodemographic characteristics have been associated with both preoperative disturbance and postoperative depression (Lalinec-Michaud & Engelsmann, 1984). This has been explained in relation to the better preparation of middle class, better educated women, and their greater understanding of the need for the surgery. It also may reflect fewer options for non-childbearing-related lifestyles and roles for these lower socioeconomic women than for middle class women. The same variables appear to affect responses to menopause (Notman, 1979).

The actual experience with the surgery itself is not often considered in evaluating the outcome. The importance of preparation, the relationship to the surgeon, the availability of supportive individuals and absence of complications affect the result.

Sexual consequences of hysterectomy have generally been linked to the vaginal dryness resulting from diminished estrogens if oöphorectomy is performed as well. Many women do report some sexual changes and a perception that the vagina is shortened. Raphael (1976) studied postoperative sexual adjustment. She reports that 30 percent of the patients in her study said they had considerable improvement, 20 percent were unchanged, and 16.5 percent were worse. The variables of significance were: Women with a bad outcome were more likely to have had abdominal hysterectomy, those with a good outcome were more likely to have had a vaginal hysterectomy. Oöphorectomy was more likely to be done during the abdominal procedure. Those who did well had been able to express concerns and hopes, and had more support. These findings are similar to those in other studies. The women with marginal sexual adjustment and less secure feminine identity experienced the surgery as a further assault to an already shaky self-image.

The pervasive implications of the procedure can also be surmised by attention to colloquial terms for it. Some women say "I lost my nature"; others describe the operation as "being cleaned out," "having everything removed." A group of Chinese women (Tsoi, Ho, & Poon, 1984) interviewed pre- and postoperatively were relieved to have had the surgery, but 70 percent of them reported a belief that "a hole would be left in the body," and 60 percent of them worried about aging.

ABORTION

Many myths have developed about the experience of abortion. It has been practiced for centuries and in many cultures. In the United States, regulation of abortion was initially instituted in the mid-nineteenth century to protect patients from careless procedures resulting in high morbidity and mortality.

The controversy concerning abortion has renewed claims that it is a psychologically damaging procedure (Pasnau, 1972). This view was prevalent before 1960; the expectations were that guilt and shame resulting from abortion would lead to serious depression and disturbances in relationships. Guilt and shame as a reaction to having an abortion were confused with reactions to committing a socially stigmatized and usually illegal act. The myth of inevitable psychological damage persisted, despite evidence to the contrary, including the results reported from Ekblad's (1955) study of 479 women who had legal abortions in Sweden for psychiatric reasons, which provided evidence that abortion was not necessarily detrimental to emotional health. Later more carefully performed research further documented this finding.

A 1969 review by the Group for the Advancement of Psychiatry (GAP, 1969) noted the lack of serious postabortion psychological complications and recommended that during the preabortion period, motivation for the decision should be explored and counseling provided when indicated. Others also emphasized the need to clarify motivation for their termination of pregnancy (American Psychiatric Association, 1970). Evidence has accumulated indicating that it is not possible to predict which women will suffer from emotional disturbances if therapeutic abortion is denied, since the reasons for not wanting a particular pregnancy have not been clearly differentiated from the manifestations of emotional stress (Sloane, 1969; Whittington, 1970).

In a 1976 report (Payne, Kravitz, Notman, & Anderson, 1976) that developed and validated scales to measure anxiety, depression, anger, guilt, and shame preabortion and postabortion, the investigators found that the pattern of response was similar to that of other instances of crisis reaction and crisis resolution. Those women who were most vulnerable to conflict following abortion were those with (1) a previous history of mental illness or serious emotional conflict; (2) immature personal relationships or unstable, conflictual relationships with men; (3) negative relationships with their mothers; (4) strong ambivalence or uncertainty and helplessness with regard to abortion; and (5) religious or cultural background in which there were negative attitudes toward abortion. In addition, single women, especially those who had not borne children, were more susceptible to conflict following abortion. The study cautioned, however, that these factors were not to be interpreted as contraindications to abortion. They pointed out that at their six-month follow-up evaluation, women in the vulnerable groups believed that their decision for abortion was the right one. The study concluded that the opportunity to play an active role in resolving the crisis of an unwanted pregnancy and to choose or reject abortion promotes successful adjustment and maturation. Thus, rather than making a decision for or against abortion on tenuous grounds, the woman seeking an abortion may benefit from a variety of crisis-intervention and therapeutic techniques. Evidence for long-term negative consequences requiring treatment does not exist.

An important aspect of this issue, one which is rarely addressed and on which there are currently few substantive data, is the outcome of alternatives to abortion, such as having the unwanted baby. Comparative longitudinal studies of women making different choices are necessary to adequately evaluate this complex factor.

At present, abortion is rarely regarded as "therapeutic," but it is seen as a matter of choice with multiple alternatives. The response is variable but involves some recognition of the loss, some working through of the crisis aspects and is usually not a major trauma, although for some women it serves to focus unresolved psychological issues and problems in relationships. It is not inconsistent also for the woman to have a positive response to the knowledge that she can become pregnant even though the decision is made to abort.

CONCLUSION

Recent research has contributed to understanding and has changed views of the effects of some gynecological procedures, such as hysterectomy and abortion. Nevertheless surgery involving the genitals and reproductive organs involves highly significant organic and psychological functions with potential major implications.

REFERENCES

American Psychiatric Association. (1970). Position statement on abortion. *American Journal of Psychiatry, 126,* 1554.

Barnes, B. (1981). An overview of hospital gynecologic practice. *Primary Care, 8,* 165–176.

Bunker, J. P., Donanue, V. C., Cole, P., & Notman, M. (1976). Elective hysterectomy, pro and con. *New England Journal of Medicine, 295* (5), 264.

Ekblad, K. (1955). Induced abortion on psychiatric grounds. *Acta Psychiatric Scandinavica Supplementum, 99,* 1–238.

Fox, R. (1957). Training for uncertainty. In R. Merton, G. Reader, & P. Kendall (Eds.), *The Student Physician* (p. 207). Cambridge, MA: Harvard University Press.

Fox, R., & Lief H. (1963). Training for detached concern in medical students. In H. Lief, V. Lief, & N. Lief (Eds.), *The Psychological Basis of Medical Practice* (p. 12). New York: Harper & Row.

Gath, D., & Cooper, P. (1982). Psychiatric disorders after hysterectomy. *Journal of Psychosomatic Research, 25,* (5), 347–355.

Gath, D., Cooper, P., & Day, A. (1982). Hysterectomy and psychiatric disorder: I. levels of psychiatric morbidity before and after hysterectomy. *British Journal of Psychiatry, 140,* 335–350.

Goldwyn, R. (1978). The woman and esthetic surgery. In M. Notman & C. Nadelson (Eds.), *The Woman Patient (Vol. 1, pp. 271–280).* New York: Plenum.

Group for the Advancement of Psychiatry. (1969). *The Right to Abortion: A Psychiatric View,* (75), pp. 197 – 227, NY Mental Health Materials Center.

Janis, I. (1958). *Psychological Stress.* New York: Wiley.

Kestenberg, J. (1961). Menarche. In S. Lorand & S. Schneer (Eds.), *Adolescents: Psychoanalytic Approach to Problems and Therapy.* New York: Hoeber.

Lalinec-Michaud, M. & Engelsmann, F. (1984). Depression and hysterectomy: A prospective study. *Psychosomatics, 25* (7), 550–558.

Lerner, H. (1976). Parental mislabeling of female genitals as a determinant of penis envy & learning inhibitors in women. *Journal of American Psychoanalytic Association, 24* (5), 269–283.

Lindeman, E. (1941). Observations on psychiatric sequelae to surgical operations in women. *American Journal of Psychiatry, 98,* 132–137.

Mazor, M. (1984). Emotional reactions to infertility. In M. Mazor & H. Simons (Eds.), *Infertility,* (pp. 23–35). New York: Human Sciences Press.

Meikle, S. (1977). The psychological effects of hysterectomy. *Canadian Psychology Review, 18,* 128–144.

Moore, N., & Tolley, D. (1976). Depression following hysterectomy. *Psychosomatics, 17,* 86–89.

National Center for Health Statistics. (1980). Utilization of short stay hospitals. In *Annual Summary for the United States,* 1980 Series, *13* (64).

Notman, M. (1979). Midlife in women; finiteness and expansion. *American Journal of Psychiatry, 136* (10), 1270–1274.

Notman, M., & Nadelson, C. (1978). The woman patient. In M. Notman & C. Nadelson (Eds.), *The Woman Patient,* (Vol. 1, pp. 1 – 7). New York: Plenum.

Pasnau, R. (1972). Psychiatric complications of therapeutic abortion. *Obstetrics and Gynecology, 40,* 252–256.

Payne, E., Kravitz, A., Notman, M., & Anderson, J. (1976). Outcome following therapeutic abortion. *Archives of General Psychiatry, 33,* 725–733.

Raphael, B. (1976). Psychiatric aspects of hysterectomy. In J. Howells (Ed.), *Modern Perspectives in the Psychiatric Aspects of Surgery* (pp. 422–446). New York: Brunner/Mazel.

Richards, T. H. (1974). A post-hysterectomy. *Lancet, 2,* 983–985.

Roeske, N. (1978). Hysterectomy and other gynecological surgery: A psychological view. In M. Notman & C. Nadelson (Eds.), *The Patient* (Vol. 1, pp. 217–231). New York: Plenum.

Sloane, R. (1969). The unwanted pregnancy. *New England Journal of Medicine, 22,* 1206–1213.

Tsoi, M. Ho, P. C., & Poon, R. (1984). Preoperation indicators and post-hysterectomy outcome. *British Journal of Clinical Psychology, (23),* 151–152.

U.S. Bureau of the census. (1982). *Statistical Abstracts of the U.S. 1982–1983,* 103rd edition, Washington D.C.

Whittington, H. (1970). Evaluation of therapeutic abortion as an element of preventative psychiatry. *American Journal of Psychiatry, 126,* 1224–1229.

Zilbach, J. (1983) (personal communication).

CHAPTER EIGHT

Psychological Adaptation to Renal Disease and Transplantation

SAMUEL H. BASCH, M.D.

With few exceptions, patients facing kidney transplantation have already had psychological confrontations with renal disease and its various treatments (Abram, 1968; Guillidge, 1983; & Kemph, 1966). Although traumatic in any age group, the untoward effects of this situation are often seen to an exaggerated degree in the young or adolescent. Inexperience and innocence allow for a florid expression of symptoms in the preadult. Disease and treatment intertwine with ongoing maturation and magnify both the problems of the adolescent and the dilemma of the uremic.

It is necessary to keep in mind that certain individuals were stricken with their disorders in childhood, and by the time they arrive at adolescence they have been suffering for a number of years. There is a wide range of variation in coping with and adapting to this specific renal situation, a situation which resembles certain medical situations yet is at variance with others (Blacher & Basch, 1970). They may have suffered retarded growth and development, with accompanying personal and social consequences, selective physical arrest or disfigurement, and a sense of chronicity or limited curability.

Whether the disease began in childhood or not, ambivalent dependency relationships are created with family and medical people. Fears may arise in the patient from the undependability of his own body — fragile, weak, and unpredictable in its metabolic instability. Patients are insecure after exposure to the vicissitudes of the underlying disease and its treatments. There is a fear of the limits of support they can receive from family, friends, and professional relationships to help them through this tribulation.

The role of loss in these young individuals is central. In addition to the loss of body intactness, other losses are legion (Basch, 1973b). Nephrectomy and inability to urinate contribute to the sense of loss of body integrity and physiologic functioning. There is an interference with drinking and eating functions. Interruptions of school attendance retard academic progress and schoolmate relationships. Disruption of athletic and recreational activities occurs. Surgery, hospitalization, and treatment cause separation from family and friends and threaten damage to or loss of important relationships (Rabinowitz, 1980). There is a giving up of the ability to plan, the loss of predictability of the future, the diminution of healthy functioning, and ultimately the fear of loss of life.

Physiologic imperatives force adolescents to confront changes in their body. They often compare their pubescence to that of their contemporaries. They are concerned with the development of new powers and skills and the ability to attract or be attracted to members of the opposite sex. Girls are concerned about breast development and menstruation. Boys are concerned about genital development, deepening voices, and facial hair. There are preoccupations with diet, acne, and weight. All of these concerns are affected, if not magnified, by renal disease and its treatments.

Both young and older individuals must deal with the changes in their body wrought by renal disease and its treatments (Cramond et al., 1968). Changes in the patient's external appearance, and internal anatomic changes and physiology, are generally profound and usually have to be dealt with at the conscious level. There are visible and profound changes sometimes with acute physiologic shifts that may unhinge the individual. A patient may find his familiar body suddenly strange in appearance, reacting in unfamiliar ways, which he experiences as "not himself." This may be fraught with a physical as well as a psychological disequilibrium, which may cause alterations in intrapsychic functioning and behavior and externally expressed personality.

Both body image and closely related self-image are affected. The way a patient feels about himself is influenced by the emphasis on his physical being and on renal treatment regimens which may severely restrict diet (water, protein, sodium intake, etc.), require myriad medications and impose on him hemodialysis or peritoneal dialysis which may occupy a significant portion of his week. The demands of the treatment interfere with family and social relationships as well as other domains of functioning. A cycle begins in which the illness and treatment dominate his life routines, internal equilibrium, affective existence, and even exaggerate the expression of certain personality traits. This, in turn, affects his behavior and external life, including his integration of the demands of his medical situation. Not unlike patients with other medical conditions (Blacher & Basch, 1970), these patients often express feeling themselves different. Some regard themselves as pariahs, misfits, or rejects. Others experience self-pity and denigration. Still others regress to a position where they regard themselves as helpless and dependent beyond what the reality dictates. Despite the severity of the illness and the extreme untoward physical and psychological effects of renal disease and its grim complications, it is the manner in which individuals cope which determines their view of themselves and their ultimate level of adaptation (De Nour, 1980).

Many patients develop fears related to the body. In addition to the dread of physical deterioration and actual death, somatic fears preoccupying many individuals can be divided into three categories: (1) external disfigurement, (2) alterations in internal body parts or organs, and (3) changes in physiology or somatic functioning.

A focus on external appearance may begin early in renal disease initiated by subtle fluid accumulation. Later the patient may feel marked by the access site (fistula, shunt) which may stigmatize him or become invested with personal meaning. One patient hid his access site so that it could not be mistaken for the "tracks" of a "junkie." One woman pressed her access site closely to her abdomen "for protection" for months following the transplantation. Some patients carried hemostats as a protection against exsanguination. After receiving several access procedures, scarred areas become a cause for concern and a focus for feelings of unattractiveness.

A sense of internal alteration can be caused by uncomfortable hemodialysis or peritoneal dialysis procedures. Nephrectomy may lead to a sense of loss, inadequacy, or incompleteness. All of these procedures may lead the patient to develop perceptions of overt or subtle physiologic changes that cannot be ignored.

With this built in body focus, it is not surprising that such patients utilize the body as a medium for expressing feelings of intrapsychic conflict. In the patients observed, three responses were noted, all of which utilized some form of denial with a somatic avenue of expression. One such response was manifested through the adoption of a "phantom kidney." An example is a nephrectomized patient who developed sensations of bladder fullness and an urge to urinate when he passed a men's room. Listening to water flush would affect him similarly. A nephrectomized woman became aware of a regression to pre-toilet training feelings, that is the sense that she had the capacity to urinate but had just not mastered bladder control. Following her transplantation, she felt tempted to "brag" to her mother that she had urinated all by herself—and that she could have all along if only she had mastered sphincter control.

A second form of response was denial of the need for an external device, by extending the body boundaries and including the dialysis machine as part of the body image. While being dialyzed one patient stated, "I'm divided in two. My blood is out there and the rest of me is back here." She further related that formerly her menstruation had served to cleanse her body but now the machine performed that function for her and did the cleaning.

Certain patients with conflicts concerning mastery may develop specific disturbance (Blacher & Basch, 1970) when they first include the dialyzer in their body scheme and then fear being controlled by the apparatus. Another way of denying the need for an external device was seen by minimizing its mechanical aspects and endowing it with human qualities. One patient referred to it as a "blood brother." Another patient said of the dialysis apparatus, "I don't like its looks. Like, sometimes you see a person and you just don't want to be involved with him." Some patients refer to the machines affectionately or feel literally and figuratively attached to the machine which is tying them down. There are references to being trapped by their body needs and the forced leaning on the medical staff and machine. One expressed, "I can't go away. I'm locked to the kidney machine, and I'd rather be dead." Several patients stricken with trapped feelings attempted to deny their dependency by insisting on taking distant trips, missing or minimizing the importance of their treatment visits, or appearing cavalier about their restrictions.

A third form of denial was manifested as an attempt to diminish the severity of the situation and to ignore the indispensibility of dialysis for survival. This was seen in the mishandling of diets, in the neglect of shunts or the patient ignoring essential routines or engaging in self damaging activities (Basch & Hartley, 1970). A number of indirect suicides may fall into this category of patients (Abram, Moore, & Westervelt, 1971).

Solidifying denial as an ongoing mechanism in the dialysand is a tenuous task since there are constant external challenges to this unsteady ego defense. Attempts at denial are interfered with by bodily sensations, weakness and malaise, or changes in physiology that may betray a movement toward an intact body image and identity. The development of confidence in the patient's physical self is also interfered with by problems in sexual functioning. This is a particular problem in patients struggling with concerns over decreased libido, impotency, infertility, amenorrhea, or decreased sexual activity (Levy, 1973).

By the time the patient is ready for transplantation, he may be disheartened by the duration or repetitive nature of hemodialysis, by the restriction of physical activities, weakness, or by complications, such as peripheral neuropathy or renal osteodystrophy. He may have had to relocate his residence, change jobs, adjust to a lower income, and alter his basic routines, diet, and life habits. Malaise may arise from his general physical condition, uremia, the treatment and its complications, and psychological enervation. He has to adopt a new identity which includes his hemodialysis and transplant experiences and has to accept new dependencies on family, medical staff, and medical technology.

A preponderance of patients facing organ transplantation at some point experience a certain degree of depression characterized by a lowering of spirits and a reduction in self-esteem. Depression observed in the transplantation patients was often precipitated by external factors, such as the treatment, complications, or the previously referred to alterations in life circumstances, and was viewed as being related to a loss of self-esteem.

Self-esteem can be defined as the value the individual finds in himself, contributed to by early life experiences and influenced by later life experiences. It includes the sexual and aggressive investment as well as the confidence one places in oneself. Self-esteem can be damaged when one does not live up to one's goals (ego ideal), whether derived from the view of one's capabilities and assets (ego potentials) as inadequate or from a demanding or oppressive sense of conscience (superego).

Self-esteem is directly affected by self-image, which is in turn affected by body image. Few psychiatrists challenge Freud's proposal that the ego is primarily a body ego. It can also be stated that, in a sense, one may view oneself as one views one's body. A sound body promotes assertiveness in life activities, whereas a fragile or sick body may lead to feelings of diffidence or insecurity. The constant abuses transplantation patients encounter, the physiologic insecurities to which they are exposed, and the intrusions on their body boundaries challenge their sense of body and in turn their sense of self.

In normal psychological development, healthy experiences during the formative years lead to a consistent and consolidated self-image that can withstand the ordinary challenges from the environment. However, the self-image is constantly undergoing minor revisions in response to environmental influences. It stands as a durable entity unless exposed to a formidable challenge. Such a challenge is seen in the extraordinary body intrusions and abuses in the transplantation situation. An assault on the body image is ultimately an assault on the self-image and can lead to dire consequences including damaged self-esteem leading to serious depression.

There are specific factors in the transplantation experience that may unfavorably affect self-esteem and lead to depression. Feelings of inadequacy brought about by difficulty in realizing occupational goals, dependency on family or medical staff, altered sexual functioning, or other unrealized or frustrated interests can damage self-regard and lead to a basic sense of inferiority. Not being able to function as previously in family, occupational, or sexual roles can lead to feelings of unworthiness. The frustrations of the dependency and passive position can lead to resentment of the caretakers (family and medical staff) with resultant guilt and self-deprecation. The sense of one's body being incomplete, altered, or mutilated contributes to feelings of being unattractive and unloved and not held in high regard. It may also lead to fears of having no one interested in oneself and of being abandoned and alone and therefore not in a position to have emotional needs met. The restrictions of the situation may make the individual feel he cannot mobilize to seek out the satisfactions he requires. These restrictions of the transplantation situation and the alterations in his life adaptation depriving him of the free reign of choices he previously enjoyed may mean he will be frustrated in having his needs gratified or in achieving his life goals. He may then conceive of himself as unsuccessful or as a failure. All these factors contribute to a poor sense of self and damaged self-esteem.

In addition to the profound effects on the renal patient from renal disease and its pretransplantation treatment (Abram, 1968; Retan & Lewis, 1966; Shreiner, 1960), the transplantation itself has specific and profound psychological effects on the individual (Basch, 1973a). One of the striking elements of the transplantation is the effect of the preceding real or fantasized relationship between the organ donor and the transplantion recipient. These patients can be considered in two categories: the recipients of family-donated kidneys and recipients of cadaver kidneys. Although there are many similarities between the two groups, there are also significant differences. The recipient of a family-donated kidney enters the transplantation situation with the cumulative complexities of the preceding relationship. Since only consanguineous relatives are donors, elements of the family drama may be compounded by the new factors in the transplantation situation.

The recipient of the cadaver kidney, on the other hand, has no previous relationship with the donor. The inert quality of the cadaver, however, offers ample opportunity for the recipient to fantasize about the donor or to transfer preconceived attitudes and feelings onto the cadaver or its organ. In addition, the recipient's associations to the lifeless state of the donor can affect his integration of the new organ.

The adjustment of the recipient of a parental kidney is influenced by the parent's and the recipient's personalities and attitudes and by the shifting relationship between the patient and the parental donor.

Case 1

Ina, a 25-year-old married female, while awaiting her transplant stated that she felt happy about receiving her mother's kidney: "My mother is a part of me. If my kidney was from a stranger, it would be like borrowing it from somebody." Although dependent on her mother, she had gone to a distant college.

The mother donor preoperatively described her feelings: "When a baby is sick you can always do something. You can give her something. With my daughter, I was helpless, and then I finally discovered and thought of an idea of doing something for her to save her life." She added that she was waiting for the time when she "would be able to give her life." When the mother was asked how she felt about being a donor, she replied: "How do you think I felt when I carried her for 9 months? She is part of me. She shared things with me then and she'll share them now." She ambivalently added, "Please, God, don't let her body reject it." The mother prepared herself for the operation by taking vitamins for the first time since her pregnancies. She believed the patient would never have become ill if she had not gone away to college but remarked, "You can't tie a child to you when they grow up."

The mother suffered a postoperative depression, was despondent, and angry. She contrasted her experience with her postpartum experience:

She was surprised and disappointed to have so much postoperative pain; the only thing she had delivered was a kidney (not a baby), with nothing to show for her suffering except a scar. On the first postoperative day the mother, weak from surgery, managed to call her daughter on an intra-hospital telephone and deliver an angry tirade. The telephone had to be disconnected to protect the daughter from her mother's invective. The mother stated: "I would give up my mind for Ina. I would give anything to make her well, but how much of nothing am I supposed to be? I've done things for my children and my husband and nobody seems to care anything about me." She added, "If something ever happens to me, they would cut me into pieces and throw me to the wolves."

Following the transplant, the patient went to great lengths to deny her dependency on the doctors. She would come to clinics late, leave quickly, and take trips to distant places. She appeared at the follow-up clinic insisting that she did not care to discuss her plan to adopt a baby and then proceeded to institute the adoption arrangements.

Psychodynamics peculiar to the maternal donor were reflected in her identification of the surgery with pregnancy: her preparing and planning, including the taking of vitamins, her sharing of organs with the offspring, her disfigurement, the giving of life, and her loss of internal contents. Although a comparison can be drawn between a postpartum reaction and the mother's postoperative anger and ambivalence, the dissimilarity may actually be the critical factor. The mother suffered a loss of a significant organ but did not bear the fruit of her pains. She felt resentment over her lack of compensation for her sacrifice. The difference between childbirth and transplantation became real to the mother only after the trans-plantation. The altruistic motivations of a maternal donor may be sincere and in keeping with the motherly role. However, beneath the surface the donor's expectation may be contrary to the reality. The unconscious factors must be carefully considered in understanding donor motivation.

Case 2

Richard, a 26-year-old prospective recipient, lived at home with his nurturing mother who was his confidante and constant companion. She even accompanied him to his only outside activity, bowling. When inter-viewed the mother volunteered a comparison to parturition by stating, "I gave birth to Richard. Now I'm giving him something of myself. I'm giving him a new start in life again. It's glorious." However, ambivalence was reflected in her covert assault through the medium of "joking" with her son about the impending transplant with statements, such as "Treat me good or I won't give you my kidney" or "A 45-year-old woman's kidney is better than none." She told him of an older man she knew "who received a kidney from a 19-year-old that made him younger." Despite this, both mother and son regretted that they could not be with each other postoperatively to give comfort to each other, and each expressed concern over being apart too long. Both Richard and his mother appeared to consider transplantation as a legitimate opportunity to intensify the pre-existing symbiosis and dependency.

In the two cases presented, the mothers expressed strong desires to continue the mother–child nurturing relationship. However, the ambivalence was marked by a posttransplantation telephone tirade in the first case and by joking threats in the second. Ina, before the transplantation, appeared to agree to the donor's rather symbiotic terms, but after the surgery she rejected her mother's attempts to rekindle an earlier dependent relationship. She strove to ensure her independence by distant travel and her plan to adopt a baby. In Richard's case, the symbiotic and dependency elements superseded the ambivalence.

A similar situation in which the kidney was endowed with unacceptable introjected qualities of the donor can be seen in the following case.

Case 3

Henry, a 10-year-old, died prior to the time the psychiatrist became a part of the transplantation program. (The information in this case came from other members of the transplantation team.) The boy initially refused to accept his father as donor because he had abandoned the family when the patient was younger. Without the boy's knowledge, the father, who professed remorse for his previous behaviour, donated the kidney that was transplanted into his son. The recipient did well until 6 months later when his father appeared unexpectedly and revealed that he was the source of the transplanted kidney. Several days later the patient was rushed to the hospital moribund; he died of severe leukopenia, explained by the doctors as secondary to an overdose of the immuno-suppressant being used.

In this case the rejecting father, attempting to make amends, imposed himself on the patient in the form of the kidney. The boy may have inadvertently ended his own life in attempting to reject his father by destroying the kidney. The organ appeared to be treated by the recipient as the personification of the donor, the hostility toward the donor being expressed against the kidney. The psychodynamics resemble those Freud proposed in explaining depression (Freud, 1917), namely, aggression toward the ambivalently conceived introjected object. The distinctive element here is the intrapsychic representation of one organ of a person (the kidney) being equated with the introjected representation of the entire person (donor).

Complexities are also seen in the sibling donor–recipient relationship. The specific conflicts exhibited in the parental donor situation were not as marked in the sibling group although other conflicts were noted. The following case illustrates the unacceptability of what the new organ can represent.

Case 4

Arnold, a 15-year-old boy, had two kidney transplantations performed at another institution but was followed up at the Mount Sinai Medical Center. The patient discussed how disturbing it had been to receive his first transplantation from a man who had shot himself. After 6 months the kidney was rejected. The second kidney was donated by the patient's 26-year-old brother. The patient described his anxiety and guilt prior to the second operation and his fear that his brother's kidney would fail and he, the patient, would die. Following the transplant, the patient did well for over a year and a half, but one morning reported to the clinic in a panic, demanding that the surgeons removed his brother's kidney. He stated that his brother was a homosexual and he did not want a homosexual's kidney inside him. Furthermore, he was dissatisfied with the kidney because his blood urea nitrogen was elevated and he feared he would die. After lengthy discussions, he agreed to keep the kidney. Following this incident, he went on a stringent diet and lost 40 pounds, saying that he wanted to be in better shape, since he was too soft and round; he wanted to feel and appear stronger, especially for the girls at school.

The patient's identification with the homosexuality of his brother was accompanied by overwhelming anxiety. Defensive attempts at resolution were made through actual changes in body appearance. The brother's kidney was conceptualized by the patient as a genitourinary introject which he first dealt with by demanding its removal; later he attempted to alter the feminine image by creating a leaner, more masculine external appearance.

Although dependency conflicts and ambivalence were more striking in the cases with parental donors, they were not absent in the sibling donor situation. The problems of cross-, or even same sex, transplantation in siblings require further study.

Just as the recipients of family donated kidneys appear to ascribe traits of the donor to the new kidney, so in a sense do recipients of cadaver kidneys, despite the absence of a previous relationship with the donor.

In the following case the father of a 17-year-old boy, was evaluated as a potential donor.

Case 5

As a child, James had made interminable but unsuccessful efforts to be closer to his remote and passive father. The father was disqualified as a donor when found to be hyperglycemic, much to the son's disappointment and simultaneous relief. James felt guilty, as if he himself had caused the diabetes by necessitating the father's transplant evaluation.

Although the patient had been informed of his prospective transplantation several weeks prior to the procedure, he was told 48 hours before the operation that "a man down the hall" was terminal and that as soon as the man died he could have his kidney. The patient prayed the entire preoperative night that the dying man might live. He felt like a "vulture," and spontaneously referred back to having felt guilt over his father's hyperglycemia. After the operation, he became curious about the donor and was told the donor's name was Jaime. He began studying Spanish, at first on his own, eventually requesting a tutor. He also imagined that the donor looked just like his uncle, for whom he had warm feelings. When he later suffered a rejection crisis and was informed that he would lose the kidney, he tearfully said, "Doctor, you'll never know just how attached I was to that kidney."

This case illustrates the patient's conflict in taking an organ from someone for personal benefit and also the recipient's struggle to integrate the foreign organ into his body image. There were pretransplantation guilt feelings about his father as a donor as well as about the actual dying donor. In his fantasy following the operation, the cadaver was not viewed as his father but as a noncontroversial and warm figure, James' uncle. He identified with only a single and neutral trait of the donor — his language.

He suffered no apparent guilt postoperatively and more easily accepted an organ to which he had become literally and figuratively attached.

In the case of cadaver kidney transplantation presented, the recipients' attitudes toward the cadaver and his organ seemed to affect their integration of the organ. Just as the recipients of family-donated kidneys appear to endow the new kidney with traits of the donor, so in a sense do recipients of cadaver kidneys, despite the absence of a previous relationship with the donor. Since there is no dynamic interaction as in the live donor situation, there is only a "taking in" of qualities. The cadaver donor is not present to serve as a reminder of dependency, indebtedness, or other conflicts, and the recipient does not have to contend with the donor's reaction to sacrificing his organ. The donor's being dead and unknown, therefore, paves the way for an intense elaboration of fantasies which, in turn, may be colored by the recipient's previous beliefs about death and dying. They are imposed on the feeling of death attached to the organ the recipient now has within him.

CONCLUSION

Young and adult individuals are affected by the transplantation and its attendant problems and losses. The data suggest how the attitudes a recipient develops toward his or her new kidney can affect the way the organ is accepted and integrated into body image. This assimilation is affected not only by the patient's preoperative ego functioning and object relations, particularly if there is a live donor, but also by the specific transplantation experience and other reality factors. In some of our patients, psychic conflict concerning the new kidney and donor appeared to contribute to physiologic changes, possible transplant rejection and, in at least two cases, death. Understanding these conflicts may help to clarify criteria predicting success or failure in potential transplant patients.

Preexisting family conflicts in the consanguineous recipients were heightened by the transplantation. Specific dyadic relationships reflected particular psychodynamic patterns, such as the dynamics comparable to those of parturition exhibited in the mother donor–child recipient cases or homosexual conflicts. Recipients of cadaver kidneys seemed affected by their fantasies about the cadaver and their attitudes toward death and dying and the lifeless, inert traits of the unknown donor. Although most transplantation patients make a satisfactory adjustment, some have serious difficulties integrating the new organ into their body image.

Although all patients have difficulty dealing with renal transplantation, conflicts in the young are magnified. The role of loss and change is profound. The connections between body image and self-image become more evident and disturbing. There are several types of body insults and losses that affect the intrapsychic mechanism of denial and other defenses. Commonly found depression affects self-esteem. The vicissitudes of integrating a new organ and the relationship between the donor and the recipient can have a profound effect on the individuals and on the outcome of the renal transplantation.

REFERENCES

Abram, H. S. (1968). The psychiatrist, the treatment of chronic renal failure, and the prolongation of life. *American Journal of Psychiatry, 124*(10), 1351–1358.

Abram, H. S., Moore, G.L., & Westervelt, F. W. (1971). Suicidal behavior in chronic dialysis patients. *American Journal of Psychiatry, 127,* 1199–1204.

Basch, S. H. (1973a). The intrapsychic integration of a new organ. *Psychoanalytic Quarterly, 42,* 364–384.

Basch, S. H. (1973b). Damaged self esteem and depression in organ transplantation. *Transplantation Procedures, 5*(2), 1125–1127.

Basch, S. H., & Hartley, J. (1970). Nineteen fractures in an accident prone patient. Psychiatric and orthopedic considerations. *Journal of Mount Siani Hospital, 371.*

Blacher, R. S., & Basch, S. H. (1970). Psychological aspects of pacemaker implantation. *Archives of General Psychiatry, 22,* 319–323.

Cramond, W. A., Knight, P. R., Lawrence, J. R., Higgins, B. A., Court, J. H., MacNamara, F. M., Clarkson, A. R., & Miller, C. O. J. (1968). Psychological aspects of the management of chronic renal failure. *British Medical Journal 1,* 539–543.

DeNour, A. K. (1980). Quality of life of dialysis and transplantation patients. *Nephron, 25*(3), 117–120.

Freud, S. (1917[1915]). Mourning and melancholia. *Standard Edition, 14,* 243–258.

Guilledge, A. D., Buszta, C., & Montague, D. K. (1983). Psychosocial aspects of renal transplantation. *Urological Clinic of North America, 10*(2), 327–335.

Kemph, J. P. (1966). Renal failure, artificial kidney and kidney transplant. *American Journal of Psychiatry, 122,* 1270–1274.

Levy, N. B. (1973). Sexual adjustment to maintenance hemodialysis and renal implantation. *"Transactions-American Society for Artificial Internal Organs," 19,* 138–143.

Rabinowitz, J. (1980). Psychological adaptations to a renal dialysis and transplantation program. *International Journal of Rehabilitation Research, 3*(1), 73–75.

Retan, J. W., & Lewis, H. Y (1966). Repeated dialysis of indigent patients for chronic renal failure. *Annals of Internal Medicine, 64,* 284–292.

Shriner, G. E. (1960). Mental and personality changes in the uremic syndrome. *Medical Annual, 28,* 316–320.

CHAPTER NINE

On the Role of Denial in Cancer Surgery

BERNARD C. MEYER, M.D.

Readers of psychosomatic literature who anticipate a periodic display of tables and charts will find little comfort in this presentation, for it contains neither, nor does it conform to the usual demands for strict organization and orderly consistency. On the contrary, no effort has been made to confine the following material within the boundaries of the stated subject, nor does it seem possible to do so. First, there are no precise distinctions between the psychological problems encountered in cancer surgery and those discovered in surgery in general. Second, it is not easy to exclude nonsurgical material from this presentation, nor does it seem desirable to do so, for such a narrowing of the focus would reflect a monocular point of view that is already too prevalent in current medical practice and thinking. Finally, it will be evident that no attempt has been made to embrace a systematic review of the subject, nor has the material been divided into nice compartments, each headed by a suitable label according to the anatomical location of the disease, to pre- and postoperative stages, to grades of malignancy, and so forth. Instead a generally loose and discursive style which, while lacking the systematic organization of usual scientific writing, may yet attain the intended goals of this presentation, namely, to call attention to the importance and complexities of the subject, and to stimulate interest in it beyond its limited range.

No aspect of medicine lends itself so readily to the wild play of imagination and to the extreme fluctuations of feeling as does the practice of surgery, and nowhere is the mental balance of all the participants subjected to greater stress than in the presence of cancer. Indeed the advent of that condition afflicts not only the patient himself, but his physician and the entire micro-cosm of which he is a member. To be sure, this is true of all grave illness. Thus, it has been shown that the death of a spouse from any cause is one of the most potentially stressful of commonly occurring life events, and consti-tutes a readily discernible cause of increased medical morbidity and mortality in the survivor. Experimental evidence in support of this claim has been provided by Schleifer, Keller, Camerino, and Stein (1983) who, in a pros-pective longitudinal study of the spouses of women afflicted with advanced breast cancer, have demonstrated that among their husbands lymphocyte production was significantly depressed following the death of their wives. Nor is there any need to document the emotional impact on the entire family resulting from the show of progressive cachexia of a dying parent or child.

Indeed it is probable that no word in the lexicon of medicine strikes greater terror in the human heart, with the result that with varying degrees of ingenuity, physicians and patients alike have devised a repertoire of euphemisms, synonyms, abbreviations, and foreign — often Latin — phrases, designed to bypass the dreaded word — cancer. Yet the effectiveness of such circumlocutions is, to say the least, debatable. Aired during bedside "rounds" the use of such terms as "CA," "mitotic figures," "mets," (for metastasis), and the like, may accomplish the very opposite of what is intended by adding a note of distrust and suspicion to the already mounting anxiety of the patient. Despite the closed eyes and an appearance of sleepiness or indiffer-ence, the latter may be acutely attentive to every word that is exchanged, or whispered (!), among the participants of what is sometimes known as "grand rounds." How long the procession pauses at each bed, and with what degree of animation or impatience, are details that may be carefully monitored by the patient, and interpreted, correctly or not, as indicators of clinical interest, hopefulness, pessimism, or personal appeal. Although some subjects may be gratified to be the focus of the serious discussions and repeated examinations taking place at the bedside, others may be badly demoralized by the entire business. Moreover, the hurly-burly of academic competitiveness, the zest for bibliographic one-upmanship, a passion for citing statistics, and a delight in "chewing out" a subordinate in the presence of an audience, are not especially conducive to the establishment of an atmosphere in which the sensibilities and serenity of the patient are of primary concern (Kaufman, Franzblau, & Kairys, 1956). Least of all does such a setting encourage a thoughtful concern with the question of what the patient should be told about his or her condition. A matter of supreme importance in the presence of neoplastic disease, this issue is sometimes handled more in accordance with a set policy — tell all, or tell nothing — than as a consequence of an informed recognition of the psychological complexities of the picture.

TELLING THE PATIENT

Often enough the question of what to tell the patient is not the real issue, for he may be far more aware of the "truth" than he is credited with, and consequently may be quick to recognize when he is being lied to. "In your relations with patients," wrote Henderson (1935), "you will inevitably do much harm, and this will be by no means confined to your strictly medical blunders. It will also arise from what you say and what you fail to say. But try to do as little harm as possible not only in treatment with drugs, or with the knife, but also in treatment with words, with the expression of your sentiments and emotions."

> The truth you speak does lack some gentleness
> And time to speak it in; you rub the sore
> When you should bring the plaster.
> — THE TEMPEST

Nowhere is this sentiment more relevant to medical practice than in the subject of cancer, where the very choice of words may prove to play a pivotal role. An example is provided by a man who was told by his surgeon that the recently performed operation revealed the presence of a "malignancy." At once he telephoned his family to give them the news, adding with evident relief, "Thank God it isn't cancer!" That at some level of awareness he may have realized that in seeking to support a denial of ill tidings he was playing a game of words seems not unlikely, yet it would be the height of folly to undermine that denial by explaining to him what he probably already knows, namely, that the words "malignancy" and "cancer" are synonymous. Instead it would seem wise to support him in his denial by adopting his own words until he is ready to abandon it and face the facts with whatever fortitude he can muster.

Yet the mental state of the candidate for cancer surgery is determined by considerations beyond those caused by the disease itself, considerations that apply to operations undertaken for any purpose whatever. Indeed, it is commonly recognized that the variety and intensity of the emotional reactions released by the prospect of surgery may bear little relevance to the gravity of the procedure, to the nature of the underlying condition, or to the general state of health of the patient. For many the essential scenario enacted in the surgical amphitheatre—the forced imposition of sleep on helpless and recumbent subjects, the cutting of their flesh and the mutilation of their body—prepares the way for a varied catalogue of wild fears and crazy fantasies. Granted that these do not reflect a conscious belief that they are victims of the surgeon's sadism and hostility, at some deeper level of thought considerations of reality may be swept aside and the experience may be virtually indistinguishable from the picture of the classic nightmare.

I trembling waked, and for a season after
Could not believe but that I was in hell,
Such terrible impression made my dream.
— KING RICHARD THE THIRD

Some persons, fearing that they may be poorly defended against the unwanted disclosure of secret thoughts and suppressed impulses, may dread the imposition of artificial sleep more than the operation itself. Some men, uncertain of their masculinity, may fear that the passive nature of the surgical experience may uncover wishes for homosexual surrender and "castration," while in women it may evoke fantasies of sexual assault and childbirth. Unconsciously in all subjects the experience may be "interpreted" variously as punishment, retribution, a rebirth, and so forth—fantasies that may be facilitated by a reactivation of an earlier traumatic event.

RELIVING CHILDHOOD EXPERIENCES

It is indeed remarkable how often surgical procedures performed in adult life are linked with memories of childhood operations, such as tonsilectomy. The passage of time may have done little to erase from memory recollections of some aspect of that experience: the sudden and unforseen separation from the parents, the wheeled journey into the unfamiliar operating room, the bright lights, the concealed faces, the strange and unappealing smell, the forced application of the anesthesia mask, the futile struggle, the terror and the stifled scream, and, finally, oblivion.

Granted that not every child has been subjected to such terrifying experiences, and that in the more sophisticated medical centers of today, childhood surgery has been divested of much of the foregoing crude and unfeeling practices, it is nevertheless true that the emotions and thoughts aroused by surgical operations in adulthood tend to be distillates of earlier traumatic experiences. The recognition of this has practical implications moreover for it may illumine some of the unforseen features of the mental state of the adult surgical subject. Thus, unencumbered by such early memories, some candidates for major surgery may approach the ordeal with surprising calm and fortitude, while others, burdened by life-long recollections of a childhood trauma, may face relatively minor procedures, like the drainage of an abscess, or the repair of a hernia, with a show of terror and a sense of doom which are inappropriate to the medical realities.

Indeed, in some instances such thoughts may attain the force of a conviction that the procedure will have a fatal outcome. Such certainties (which must be distinguished from a not unusual preoperative fear) are impervious to reassurances and appeals to reason. The surgeon's assertion that the patient is in excellent general health, that the operation in question enjoys a strikingly low mortality rate, and other logical arguments fall on deaf ears, for the force of the patient's belief arises not from reason but from some remote chamber of the mind where unreason holds sway. Driven by inexorable unconscious forces such patients present a challenge that may unnerve even the most confident surgeon. In fact, experienced physicians who have learned to respect the influence of unconscious mental processes on bodily function are often loath to operate in these cases, at least pending psychiatric intervention, for too many instances have been recorded in which such Cassandra-like forebodings have come true.

Psychiatric inquiry into these cases has revealed that ulterior to the prediction of an inevitable fatal outcome there often lies a conscious or an unconscious wish to die. Prompted by the quest for retribution, burdened by intolerable guilt, or oppressed by an unrelieved sense of hopelessness, some hapless persons view the hazards of surgery as a welcomed opportunity to outwit the finger of fate. An example may be seen in the case of a young man who was convinced he would not survive the incision and drainage of a lung abscess. Assured of the slight morbidity accompanying the procedure, and confronted by an impressive catalog of evidence of his general good health, he remained unmoved and unconvinced. Summoned by the surgeon, a psychiatrist discovered that ulterior to the patient's unswerving conviction lay an element of retribution, impelled by his fancied responsibility for the death of his child from pneumonia. Less dramatic than this play of the *lex talionis* (both father and child were afflicted with a pulmonary condition) are those instances in which the appeal of death is rooted in the state of chronic depression (Hackett and Weisman, 1960). For such individuals suffering from a *taedium vitae*, a guiltless alternative to suicide is provided by the surgeon's hand. It is not surprising, under the circumstances, that, thrust unwittingly into the role of executioner, an intuitive doctor may be reluctant to play his part.

Yet even in the absence of such dire pronouncements there is little doubt that emotional factors may play a crucial role on the course of surgical—as well as medical—illness. Not only the matter of survival, but the incidence of complications and the tempo of convalescence, may all be influenced by the mood and spirit of the patient—briefly put, by his will to live (Kennedy & Bakst, 1966).

It goes without saying that the impact of these issues is enlarged when they concern the matter of cancer. For now the operation deals with more than a question of treatment; it has now become an instrument of diagnosis and prognosis, an answer to an array of ominous questions concerning hopes, doubts, suspicion, and dread, as well as an introduction to images of mutilation, wasting, and death. In awaiting the answers to questions, such as: What did they find? Did they get it all? — the patient is beset by the same conflict between an unwilling acceptance of reality and an eager embrace of denial that has beleaguered him from the first signs of the illness.

DENIAL

In the face of all the present-day publicity regarding cancer, and the need for early detection and periodic checkups, it is remarkable how patently serious signs and symptoms may be ignored or explained away by sophisticated and reasonable people, not excluding physicians. Thus, many years after her menopause the appearance of bleeding from the rectum was interpreted by an intelligent woman as the return of her menses, an "interpretation" that required the denial both of her menstrual history and her knowlege of anatomy. Spurred on by the wish to ignore a sign of danger to her well-being, she was able to include yet another wish, namely, that she was still capable of bearing a child.

If wishes were horses then
Beggars would ride.
Put beggars on horseback,
And then, woe betide!

Such an antinomy between cancer and creativity is a not uncommon feature in the mental life of patients afflicted with a malignant disease. Another woman, who suffered from a paraplegia caused by spinal metastases from breast cancer, asked whether her breast would grow back, and whether she might still have another baby. This naive show of denial was evident throughout the course of her illness. From the start she had ignored the possible significance of the lump in her breast and had applied an ointment in order to make it "go away." With the progression of her disease she made no causal connection between the unsightly festering mass and her back pain and neurolgical symptoms, which she attributed to "arthritis." That at some level of awareness she may have recognized the quasi-psychotic nature of her denial is suggested by her complaint of being "nearly crazy with pain," and her assertion that one could "become insane from lying here so long." Moreover at night, she became severely agitated when she saw the shadows and figures of little men on the ceiling—they carried knives and looked like pirates.

Denial may also be effected by a paranoid displacement of dysfunction from the self to other objects. Only after a series of plumbers failed to find anything wrong with the faucets and the pipes in his house was it discovered that a patient was concealing his concern over his own urological malfunctioning.

Nor does the role of denial cease following surgery. In a study of recovery room subjects, Winkelstein, Blacher, & Meyer, (1965) found that the seeming obtundence of patients following the regaining of consciousness after surgery was more a function of psychological factors—suppression and denial—than of pharmacological ones. It was noted that despite an appearance of lucidity, during the immediate postoperative state these patients exhibited a striking lack of concern about the operative findings as well as a general absence of pronounced affective responses. After an interval, of approximately 24 hours, however, the picture changed, and the concerns and emotions that had been so conspicuously lacking a day earlier broke forth in full force. In some instances, the expected reactions may be postponed for an even longer interval.

Although following the amputation of the breast or other mutilative procedures it is natural and normal for signs of depression to appear, there are times when, far from being depressed, the postoperative patient may appear unaccountably cheerful, and even elated. In such cases, however, the appropriate reaction has merely been delayed, for the patient has devised ways to avoid a confrontation with ugly reality. Seemingly disinterested, she may avoid engaging the surgeon in an inquiry about the operation, and while her dressings are being changed she is careful to look the other way. However, once these measure are no longer feasible, her mood may swiftly change and the depression finally unfolds. In some instances, indeed, the refusal to look at the mutilated body may continue for months or longer. For over a year, a woman who had undergone mastectomy managed to avoid viewing her naked body. She took baths in the dark, and did not turn on the lights until she had concealed her disfigured body behind a housecoat.

This capacity for denial is especially impressive when it is employed by a sick physician, who, in the face of signs and symptoms whose meaning would be obvious even to a third-year medical student, succeeds in scuttling his professional knowledge in order to embrace the diagnosis of a benign condition. Thus, a clinician of national repute, confronted by all-too-obvious signs of a carcinoma of the head of the pancreas, accepted without evident question and with immense relief his surgeon's diagnosis of "hepatitis" following a bypass procedure of the biliary system. "What a fool I have been!" he exclaimed, beaming with pleasure. We are not suggesting that throughout the entire fabric of his thinking he remained ignorant of the true state of affairs, but rather that the circumstances were such as to permit him to suppress what he did not wish to comprehend. The contrived subsidence of the jaundice reinforced his capacity for denial, so that after leaving the hospital he was able to resume his practice for a time and maintain the facade of a convalescent with a good prognosis. In the course of time, to be sure, he began to fail and he recognized the deception that had been played on him with his own connivance, as it were. Opinions may vary as to the moral or philosophical questions involved here.

Despite these measures to deny an unpalatable truth, the patient's dreams often may disclose the unsubstantial or porous character of the denial. A few nights prior to surgery, the patient who "interpreted" the rectal bleeding as a return of her menses, dreamed that she was to appear on a television show where she was to sing a number entitled, "Make Believe." Similarly, not long after undergoing a total colectomy and colostomy, a young man (not a cancer patient) dreamed that he was an architect who was inspecting a cathedral. To his dismay he found that the altar had been constructed in the front, instead of at the rear of the church where it belonged. When he remonstrated with the builders he was told that it was too late and too costly to make any changes. Previously cheerful—inappropriately so—on awakening he felt deeply depressed.

The use of denial as a defense is no less evident in the dying patient, where it may take the form of preoccupation with seemingly trivial problems, like an undue concern with the care of toe nails. Yet lest this seeming distraction from the matter of dying be dismissed as mere caprice devoid of meaning, it should be noted that here, as in other cases previously cited, the function of the denial serves more than a simple avoidance of an intolerable reality, for on focusing his attention on the normal growth of a discrete part of the body, the subject succeeds not only in diverting his thoughts from the fearsome prospect of death, but in affixing them on emblems of propagation and life. A more dramatic manifestation of this pattern was displayed by a recently married 60-year-old man, who, knowingly afflicted with metastases from an incurable cancer, caused his young wife to become pregnant bearing his posthumous child. Some tombstones, notably in Asian countries, are furnished with hollowed-out drinking place for birds, signifying that life continues even in a place of death.

For each age is an age that is dying,
Or one that is coming to birth.
— ARTHUR O'SHAUGHNESSY

Just as there is much variety in the style in which people face their own death, so there is no regularity in the manner in which they endure that partial death that is implicit in bodily mutilation. It may be supposed, for example, that for a young, unmarried woman the loss of a breast or the imposition of a colostomy will elicit a different emotional response than when the same fate is visited on an older person who has felt fulfilled in her role in life as a mother and a wife. Yet despite such logical considerations the matter of mourning over the loss of body parts may transcend the questions of past achievement and injury to self-esteem. Just as surgery in the adult years may reactivate memories of earlier trauma, so may the loss of body parts in later life revive recollections of earlier losses.

A night or two after undergoing a mastectomy, a woman who had apparently "accepted" the procedure with an apparent show of equanimity, had a dream from which she awoke in a mood of melancholy. In the dream she saw herself, arms outstretched, pursuing her 9-year-old son who had died some years before. It was all very frustrating, she recalled, for as fast as she ran her boy ran even faster, so that she could never catch up with him.

When she was asked in what direction was he running, she replied, "It's funny. To the left; always to the left!" It should come as no surprise to learn that it was her left breast that had been removed.

Aside from the plausible conjecture that the dream expressed the hope that just as she had surmounted the earlier loss she would now endure the present one, it is no less justifiable to discern in it an unconscious equation between the two losses: breast and child, a fusion of self and object which may be viewed too as a restoration of the oneness implicit in the act of nursing. An analogous conception was conveyed by another patient who compared the disgust aroused by the sight of her colostomy with the sentiments a mother might feel on giving birth to a defective child.

Clearly an evaluation of the psychological impact of cancer surgery transcends such realistic issues as the grade of malignancy, the risk of metastasis, the threat of mutilation, and death. No less crucial is an understanding of its significance within the broad context of a lifetime of human relationships.

"Every inhabitant of the earth," wrote Samuel Johnson (1963), "must walk downward to the grave alone and unregarded, without any partner of his joy or grief, without any interested witnesses of his misfortunes or success." Composed within a week of his mother's death, these words may be construed as an expression of his grief, like the fictional work *Rasselas*, written in eight consecutive nights while she was dying. Yet these works were more than a literary requiem for his mother. As products of artistry and imagination they served both as a distraction from his grief and as an affirmation of the creative spirit through which he might establish a renewed contact with collective humanity. Analogous mental mechanisms may be discerned in a wide sampling of creative works in which the production of a work of art appears as a reparative antidote to illness or loss. An example may be seen in the case of the Hungarian composer Béla Bartók.

Stricken with leukemia, and languishing despondently in a hospital bed, a sudden breath of energy was bestowed on Bartók by the unexpected visit of the conductor Serge Koussevitzky, who offered him a commission to write a piece for the Boston Symphony Orchestra. The effect was electric: a day later, he was home again and "an enormous change seemed to have taken place—as if the entire centre of his being had been restored and reawakened" (Fassett, 1958).

Whether this unmistakable endorsement and acknowledgement of Bartók's creative genius affected his hematological status is conjectural. Suffice it to say that, as noted earlier, there is experimental evidence suggesting that this may be so (Schleifer et al., 1983).

Like the visit of Koussevitzky to Bartók's bedside, a pivotal role in providing the stricken patient with "a partner of his joy or grief" may be played by the physician. It has been shown that a visit to the patient prior to the operation by the anesthesiologist may exert a calming influence outweighing the sedative effect of a barbiturate (Egbert, Battit, Turndorf, & Beecher, 1963), just as a visit to the recovery room by a physician who is known to the patient may exert a steadying influence in beckoning him or her back to reality and to the world of the living (Winkelstein et al, 1965). It is indeed remarkable how pain may be relieved, anxiety tamed, and melancholy lifted by the unhurried and faithful attendance of the doctor, who, seated—not standing—by the bedside, reveals a calm willingness to listen, even to minor complaints, to answer questions, and to explain every step in the course of the illness and its treatment.

Like all disease, cancer may prove to be a pathway leading toward a further alienation of the individual from the stream of life or an avenue toward greater intimacy in human relationships. In this denouement in the patient's life in which he or she may confide dark secrets to his pillow in the lonely silence of the night, or partake freely in a poignant drama shared by his family and his friends, the physician make play a central role, a matrix around whose person suffering is shared and hopes rekindled.

How he solicits heaven,
Himself knows best; but strangely-visited people. . .
The mere despair of surgery, he cures.
— MACBETH

REFERENCES

Egbert, L. D., Battit, G. E., Turndorf, H., & Beecher, H. K. (1958, August 17). The value of the preoperative visit by an anesthetist. A study of doctor–patient rapport. *Journal of the American Medical Association, 185,* 553.

Fassett, A. (1958). *The Naked Face of Genius.* Boston: Houghton Mifflin.

Hackett, T. P., & Weisman, A. D. (1960). Psychiatric management of operative syndromes. *Psychosomatic Medicine, 22* (4) 267–282.

Henderson, L. K. (1935). Physician and patient as a social system. *New England Journal of Medicine. 112:* 819.

Johnson, S. (1963). The idler 41, in W. J. Bate (Ed.), *The Idler and the Adventurer* (pp. 128–131). New Haven: Yale University Press.

Kaufman, M. R., Franzblau, A. N., & Kairys, D. (1956). The emotional impact of ward rounds. *Journal of Mount Sinai Hospital, 23,* 782.

Kennedy, J., & Bakst, H. (1966). Influence of emotion on the outcome of cardiac surgery: A predictive study. *Bulletin of the New York Academy of Medicine, 42,* (10), 811–845.

Schleifer, S. J., Keller, S. E., Camerino, M., Thornton, J. C., & Stein, M. (1983). Suppression of lymphocyte function following bereavement. *Journal of the American Medical Association, 250,* 374–377.

Winkelstein, C., Blacher, R. S., & Meyer, B. C. (1965). Psychiatric observation on surgical patients in recovery room. *New York State Journal of Medicine, 65,*(7), 865–870.

— CHAPTER TEN

Becoming a Burn Victim

NORMAN R. BERNSTEIN, M.D.

Being burned differs from other experiences of illness in its abruptness and permanent change in appearance. There is a sudden turnabout — from a state of health to the condition of patienthood and dependence on medical technology. It is estimated that two million people sustain some minor burn injury each year. This includes every burned finger, each hot stove touched carelessly, or similar minor self-limited damage. It is the 100,000 people or so who enter hospitals each year because of significant thermal injury that endangers life and leaves them with permanent scarring. *First* degree burns cause minor epithelial damage to the skin, with redness and discomfort. *Second* degree burns or partial thickness burns go partially through the skin. *Third* degree or full thickness burns destroy all elements of the skin with damage going into the subcutaneous fat. All layers of the skin are destroyed, inluding nerve endings. These injuries do not leave viable skin tissue from which to regenerate epithelium and skin grafting must be carried out to cover the wound. Serious burns may damage tendons, muscle tissue, and bone.

Burn injuries are generally described in terms of the percentage of the total body area involved. We will generally discuss burns involving over 20 percent of the body area which are third degree type or greater. In such wounds, there is also some second degree burn as well. A deep burn of the face can be in a small area but significantly alter a patient's life. Third degree burns do not heal without permanent scarring. For clarity, it is useful to focus on individuals who have incurred a true accident which alters them. People who attempt suicide by immolation are different whether motives be political or psychopathological. Electrical injuries where adolescents are taking risks by climbing into dangerous areas must be left out. They often lose limbs and face the problems of amputees rather than typical burn victims. Chemical injuries and the large number of family conflicts that lead to people intentionally burning each other or recklessly producing dangerous conditions, such as unattended stoves, must be excluded as they involve an altered focus as does the arsonist who harms himself while burning down a factory for money.

We will try to get at personal experiences in previously normal and intact individuals. Allport (1942) spoke of the significance of personal documents as "any self-revealing record that intentionally or unintentionally yields information regarding the structure, dynamics, and functioning of the author's mental life" which could be helpful because he felt, citing William James, that these personal documents were the most "feasible method of approaching . . . and discovering the fundamental ways in which people came to terms with the universe."

Of the large numbers of people who sustain burn injuries each year, the general public sees few of them in ordinary daily life. Badly disfigured individuals tend to hide, and for this reason, the disfigured are a minority that are not known to the public. The suffering of its members is often kept secret and the outcomes of their lives oftan remain unknown.

People who have been significantly burned may not show visible residual symptoms which stigmatize them in public. Naturally, people try to cover their wounds. As conventional clothing can cover all but face and hands, avoidance of beach and swimming can help keep burn scars well camouflaged. These people with nonvisible scars generally do not want to talk about their problems; they repress and suppress what has happened to them. In addition, there is often traumatic amnesia for all or parts of their experience of the burn event. Burn patients sometimes say they recall that they were in the hospital for months but they do not have any memory of what happened. The amount of the material recalled relates to the age of injury. People burned early in life forget and repress more. But recall is also correlated with the context of the injury, loss of consciousness at the time, and complex individual symbolism plus repressive powers, and the overall course of injury and treatment. It bears no simple relationship to how well adjusted or disturbed the burn patient has been in the past.

About one-third of the patients hospitalized for burns have facial injuries and a large number have grossly disfigured hands. Thus, there are many people who have been burned who must live with the constant social burden of their scars, who cannot cover their disfiguration, and who remain poignantly aware of the experience that they have undergone. These people change abruptly from normal-appearing individuals to permanently different-looking individuals who are objects of what society does toward the disfigured and the handicapped. They become inhabitants of the world of the stigmatized and deviant. They contrast with the hundreds of thousands of Americans who go for cosmetic surgery each year—people who look unremarkable but feel ugly; individuals who are not regarded as abnormal looking, but who for professional, neurotic, or cultural reasons work to change their appearance toward some image they personally desire. The burn – disfigured are viewed sharply by society as ugly and unwanted. They have little choice in the matter.

FEAR

Case 1

Margaret was an energetic, eccentric, coquettish commercial artist, 48 years old, living in the Northwest. She was twice divorced. She had three grown children who lived apart. She came home one snowy night wearing a fur coat and entered the hallway of her apartment where she saw flames and smoke at one end of the hall. She stood and looked for ways to get help and there was an explosion due to faulty heating equipment. Margaret was very badly burned on her face and both hands. She was brought to a nearby hospital where intravenous fluids were started, antibiotics given, and she was transferred to a burn care centre. She recalled the shock of the explosion but no great pain.* What followed was a confused, dream-like, turbulent, timeless phase. She was isolated from people. Her eyes were covered for what seemed an eternity (actually several days according to the hospital chart). She was given drugs that dazed her. She found

---

* As third degree burns destroy the nerve endings the acute pain sensations are eradicated after the first terrible agony of being burned.

herself having hallucinations of long deceased family members and friends. Memories of her first husband recurred, as did images of her children. Plans for commercial art projects left uncompleted came drifting through her mind. As she became clearer and the delirium faded, she found her hands were in restraints. Her fingers were spread on splints so that she could not feed herself and could hardly move. Her eyes were uncovered as her discolored, swollen eyelids improved and her corneas were found undamaged. Her face was coated with thick antibiotic cream. She started hydrotherapy on another ward where she sat in a large tank and her hands were soaked and scraped every day. A week after this began, she was taken to surgery.

Her experience of going to the operating room was one of boundless terror. Margaret was sure that she would die, that she would never escape. She had images of being drawn and quartered or flayed alive, and medieval paintings were conjured up—pictures of Hieronymus Bosch, and her own fantasy drawings recurred. She underwent four repeat visits to surgery. Although she lost only one digit on her left hand, she was preoccupied with the dread sense that they were going to take off her hands each time she went to surgery.

She did not look at her face in a mirror for many weeks. It remained covered with thick white sulfa myelon cream but there was also a major effort by the staff not to let her see mirrors and not to have her examine herself closely in reflections from unused television screens. She had continued discomfort in her fingers. They ached; they were sore; and they were restrained. Going to the hydrotherapy tub and having them scraped was painful. She had never seen parts of her body scraped off. Only in menstruation had she seen her body produce blood. Her sense of her skin as the permanent boundary of herself was traumatically ruptured.

After several weeks in the hospital, Margaret became discouraged. She was visited by her children and some friends, but she felt isolated, alienated, and lost. She felt her face had been destroyed. She thought of herself as a pretty woman who had always been able to charm people and now she believed herself to be a monstrosity. She felt inconsolable in the beginning. She tried to cooperate with the procedures which were done to her, but basically, she had little choice as she felt weak and helplessly manipulated by the aides, technicians, nurses, and doctors around her.

After 16 weeks and multiple procedures including grafting of her face and scar revision, Margaret went home but kept going back to the hospital for more surgery for 2 years. In the first year after her injury, she began to draw and paint pictures of herself showing flames, a ravaged face, and ghastly disfigurement. She felt she had sustained the loss of her beauty and destruction of her inner self. These themes were painted and drawn with obsessive repetition for months. After getting out of the hospital, Margaret made firm resolutions to go back to commercial art. She produced art work for a year after she returned home, gradually doing less and less and dropping projects in the middle in a manner which she had never permitted herself before. She felt she had lost her vital energy.

Margaret became interested in religion and tried to tie some of her experiences in the isolation ward to sensations of religious transport or a feeling of being dissociated from the world that had occurred when she was submerged in artistic creation. She had been raised a Presbyterian but in adolescence had lost all religious interest and most belief. She was a vague agnostic at the time of her accident but after her hospital discharge began to search for a theological meaning for what had happened. She read the Bible every day and stopped reading newspapers or following the news on the radio or television. She took instruction from a local fundamentalist preacher but would not expose herself to going to church.

At the same time that she was exploring religious beliefs, she was spending more time at home. She feared that people would not look at her. She had her children go shopping for her. She did not keep in touch with her old friends and felt that her energies were taken up simply using her deformed hands to brush her teeth, to dress herself, and to try to make up her face. Margaret's face repelled her every time she saw it in the mirror though she tried to deal with this revulsion by making self portraits in a series hopefully intended to show improvement over the months. But these tapered off as the improvement stopped and the scars remained. She was treated by a very reserved and capable plastic surgeon and she became enormously attached to him, telling her family that she loved him but telling him only that she wanted to do a portrait of him. This she offered as a gift and she phoned him often on any pretext. His reaction was one of embarrassment and withdrawal from her, feeling that she was rather peculiar, an "artsy" lady who made him feel very uncomfortable with her sad attentiveness.

One of the events that came up a year after her accident was the suggestion that she bring suit against the building managers, the people who had constructed the building, the manufacturers of the heating equipment, and the absentee landlord who owned the building. There were mixed stories of making a fortune, of punishing the people who had harmed her, and of getting an income that would make her life easier and would pay for any further surgical care. Margaret oscillated between glorious hopes of luxury and the most modest expectations (which were actually the ones the lawyer offered) that she would get some money to cover her medical expenses. However, although the idea of a lawsuit buoyed up her spirits, consumed a good deal of her energy and focused her anger at her fate, it did not bring her further out of the house. She ultimately lost the case after intricate legal actions, and received no money. She stayed at home and conducted her affairs by telephone. She even set up a telephone code, having people ring several times and then ring back before she would pick up the phone in order to avoid social contacts, as only her lawyer, children, and selected friends knew the code. The fundamentalist church visitor continued to see her regularly at home. After years of being nonreligious, she found solace in thinking she could discern a theological meaning to what had happened to her; a reason for her catastrophe. There was a fragile sense of acceptance of her fate that came with this though overall her life was tinged with great sadness and the imprint of loss. She felt fatigued and preoccupied with dressing and feeding herself in a pattern of reclusiveness that was entrenched when she was seen 5 years later.

PAIN

Case 2

Jack, was a business man, 50 years old, whose hobby was jewelry making. As part of this work, he kept a number of inflammable solvents around. He had been working while feeling rather discouraged one evening. He had a few drinks and was careless about the Bunsen burner near the chemicals and detonated an explosion which burned him directly on the face, arms, chest, and hands and also ignited clothing, causing burns on his upper thighs. His genitilia were spared. The patient remembered the intense searing pain of his initial injury. He recalled screaming, and his wife calling the police ambulance, and being brought to the hospital with the pain disappearing. Jack reported a period of amnesia for the next 48 hours. He said that he could remember after that a hospital course of confusion, drugs, and a seemingly endless series of trips to the tub room with scraping of dead skin so that there would be no nidus for infection which would prevent the wounds from healing over.

He recalled the screaming of other patients as well as his own helpless cries and the terror with which he faced seeing bits of his flesh floating in the tub in front of him as they worked to take off more and more necrotic tissue. This was the focus of his memory flashbacks for years afterward. He feared this deep aching pain. He tried not to complain but he was always asking for more medication and felt that he did not get enough.

Jack experienced one of the great problems of burn care, the reluctance of many physicians to use narcotics. Some doctors say that good nursing care can deal with it, some emphasize hypnosis, some stress operant conditioning, pain contracting, and the use of tranquilizers but there is a general apprehension that the use of too much narcotics will lead to addiction (Perry, 1983). In reality addiction is almost unheard of in burn patients as a result of care. Concerns about addiction are derived from the drug epidemic in our society as well as vague culture bound attitudes about how much pain patients feel and how much they should bear stoically. Pain tolerance is complex and varied. Individual differences are myriad. Cultural factors are unclear. Australian and British surgeons appear to give less narcotics and consider Americans somewhat squeamish. Chinese burn surgeons give no narcotics after the first 2 days (Chi Teh Chang, personal communication, November, 16, 1983). Chinese physicians in Hong Kong use more analgesics and their patients do not behave as stoically. Jack felt that he had been cruelly abused by some of the nurses and doctors who withheld medications. The times he was in pain seemed endless. Pain care in burns is a theme going back to the descriptions of the burned Royal Air Force pilots of 1940 given in *Faces from the Fire* (Mosely, 1962) the biography of Sir Archibald MacIndoe, a brilliant pioneer burn surgeon, depicting that when the agony of dressing and debridement began they could not tell whether it lasted 5 hours or 5 years. Yet, many patients will work very hard in physical therapy in great pain to force themselves to make progress. Others surrender to the pain as Jack did, feeling helpless, despairing, and permanently shattered. Jack felt he would never come out of his experience. He felt he was never going to be human or whole again. He remained permanently less active, less social, and diminished in his work capacity feeling the scars as an unavoidable sign of inadequacy, even though facial scarring was minimal.

DEPRESSION

Depression after a burn is a regular part of the experience on the ward. These patients are relentlessly exposed to repeated dressing changes, tubbing, traction, and surgical procedures to remove dead tissue, to graft new skin, and to make revisions and reconstructive surgery for their wound sites. After 8 weeks shut up on a burn ward, they feel dejected, they are physiologically depleted, they are emotionally exhausted and time passes without their seeing a clear path to a successful return to the world. They cannot judge progress. Most surgeries seem merely further frightening events with more bandages and restraints until months have passed, and they can clearly realize that they are stronger and their wounds are covered with a new body surface albeit a rough, red one. They begin to digest the reality that they will never be the same again.

BODY IMAGE

Schilder (1950) described the body image as the changing picture in the three dimensions we have of our bodies that includes what we should look like, what we do look like, and postural knowledge about ourselves. The body image also changes when we think about ourselves on a date or at sports. One of the things that all seriously burned patients must do is to accommodate to their altered body and self-images. Wright (1960) described that in order to accept a disability, one must make changes in values; and that one must see different aspects of life available from the ones that were emphasized before the accident. She reported "containment of the effects of disability." She goes on to say that patients can epitomize themselves as "I am nothing but an incomplete, injured person who has always to mourn his loss" or a second form, "I am as I am and though I don't have all the possible assets which can be imagined, my life is full."

The burned person has grown up and been educated in a society which is determinedly focused on good looks and attractive appearance. The burn patient is not distorted or neurotic or merely defeatist when he says, "I will never look the same." This is a reality and the burn patient knows the world will not make things easy for his altered, unattractive appearance. These patients also feel that being special or unique has been submerged in their role as *burn patients*, rather than as individuals; teachers, plumbers, or spouses with burns. This dehumanization is an almost inevitable part of the hospital situation. Cousins (1981) wrote;

> "Is no penalty to be attached to a process in which a human being feels less important than the illness being diagnosed or treated? Is there nothing upsetting or even terrifying about being made to run a gauntlet of different diagnostic

faces, different instrumentations, and different procedures at a time when the last thing in the world a patient needs is more uncertainty? The medical technologist celebrates computerized tomography. The patient celebrates the outstretched hand."

In the field of burn technology, there has been enormous and life saving progress. New types of grafts, new efforts to control infection, advances in the management of shock, increased survival from larger and larger burns are all very real parts of the progress that burn medicine has made. However, almost all of them do exactly what has been described previously, they make the patient into more of a disease entity and less of a person. In the burn situation alone the emphasis on infection control—a very serious and frequently fatal problem—requires gowning, isolation units, masking, washing, and distancing from patients. The staff become anonymous behind these masks and gowns, and relatives more alien. Different institutions have varying rituals for dealing with infection but almost all of them segregate their patients behind walls, glassed or otherwise, in separate rooms away from physical contact and frequently visible contact from all of the important people in their lives. Their children are routinely kept out of the hospital altogether.

HYPNOSIS

One of the techniques that is sometimes used in the treatment of burn patients is hypnosis. Hypnosis serves a number of functions in dealing with control of pain, in dressing changes, physical therapy, and the unwillingness of burn patients to eat. One of the features that is often involved in hypnotic induction is actually touching the patient or holding an intact part of the patient. For many individuals that is, indeed, very important to them that they were physically contacted, that someone reached through the anonymity and sense of isolation to the real self of the patient.

Case 3

Robert a 25-year-old graduate student in physics was working in his laboratory when a tremendous explosion occurred in the bubble chamber in the adjoining laboratory producing an enormous fire. He fled from the building but realized there might be other people inside and ran back in and dragged out a maintenance worker who had been surrounded by flames and was unconscious. Robert sustained disfiguring burns on his face, chest, hands, and legs. He described the isolation, pain, and despair in the hospital as unbearable even though he was constantly attended by colleagues from school. His professors, fellow graduate students, and undergraduate students visited him. The faculty gave him homework and discussed physics with him to occupy him in the hospital.

Though he went through a period of depression and felt deformed and exhausted for days at a time, he believed he had links to the outside world through these individuals who kept in touch with him and enabled him to use his intact brain. He had not lost that. Still he felt the isolation, loss of control, weakness, and the vulnerability of his plight. It made him feel lost, alone, an out of contact with real life.

Part of the time he was seen by a psychiatrist who did hypnosis. This was used to help him bear the pain of dressing changes and also to eat better. He was an eagerly cooperative hypnotic subject. He wanted the technique to really "get" him and rescue him. The patient seemed dramatically helped by these procedures. Several years later at a follow-up interview, he remarked that he was still worried that when he heard the psychiatrist's voice he felt he was going into a hypnotic trance. He also remembered vividly the laying on of hands when the psychiatrist touched him on the intact surface of his arm and shoulder as part of the hypnotic induction routine. This had been a link to him that supplemented the kinds of intellectual contacts made by his colleagues. He returned to his studies and made a career as a competent and likable laboratory worker who lived an isolated life not venturing away to scientific meetings and avoiding contacts with strangers because he had several upsetting experiences of scientists becoming terrified when they beheld his scarred face.

SPECIAL CASES

Certain patients will be particularly offensive to the staff. With some patients, cursing, swearing, and letting out their feelings will be treated tolerantly by the staff. Racial and ethnic epithets aimed at personnel may be ignored for some but for other patients there may be tremendous reverberations of anger toward them. These patients can feel very much the rage of the staff that does not retaliate in terms of formal actions but sets up a negative attitude toward them. This is remembered long after by patients as the iciness of the staff. Some patients remember ruefully how difficult they were and others simply denounce the staff. On the other side, there are moral issues of a very different kind. Special patients may be favoured by a particular surgeon. This can be a concert artist who has lost all her fingers and makes the surgeon sympathetic. Some patients may be abusive and negativistic and still be cheerfully tolerated as "cute," "mischievious," or "just a kid" if their social style is an engaging one. This may be the young emergency room nurse who is very concerned after a major burn injury that she has lost her appearance and who sets up sympathetic vibrations in all the young women nurses who are caring for her. In one particular case, the injured nurse tried, in very gross ways, to deny the extent of her disfigurement and caused extreme anguish in the nursing staff, which felt a need to confront her with reality but felt they could not do so without medical consent. They did not have this and restrained themselves. They kept up a relationship with her for 2 years after she had been discharged from the hospital when the issue of her acknowledging her disfigurement was worked through in the real world, after many experiences of having to deal with a public that was put off by her scars and breached her denial.

Rowdiness, joke telling, flirting, and posturing all occur endemically in any hospital. In reports of the several hundred British assault troops and naval personnel injured in the Falkland Islands fighting, much of the same kind of joking, camaraderie, and forced cheerfulness took place that was seen in the World War II wounded and described in so many war films. This is a very useful style for maintaining group spirit and morale. An analogous group, the Israeli soldiers injured in the fighting in Lebanon had a high incidence of burn injuries inside armoured personnel carriers and tanks. Israeli military patients do not go to military hospitals (which do not exist) but rather go to civilian hospitals where they are treated as very special cases, as heroes of their country. For a young Israeli burn patient to be both petted and flirted with by nurses in spite of his disfigurement would be part of his special status (D. Gilboa, personal communication, July 1986).

Case 4

Derek, a 20-year-old Welsh guardsman was burned in the Falkland Islands when his ship Galahad was struck by an Argentine Exocet missile. He sustained 40 percent third degree burns, and 18 months after the event was in a military hospital to have a nose constructed and his hands grafted. He was grotesquely mutilated but he had been shown on national television as a hero of his country and refused to acknowledge any inner problem from his disfigurement. He said that anyone who didn't want to look at him didn't need to. "I'm all right. It's their problem, isn't it?" But he had forced his girlfriend to stop visiting and talked repeatedly of his fellow burn patients who became regularly drunk and broke up bars when out of the hospital.

All of this contrasts with civilian burn patients who are often looked on as if their own stupidity, drunkedness, or negligence had caused the accident and who are not given a great deal of admiration or sympathy. They clearly feel this in the course of their hospitalization, especially since it is added to the rejection of their disfiguration.

Many patients have flashbacks to the episode of the accident. One young worker who was inside a bricklined chamber when gas ignited had daily recurrent dreams and thoughts of being trapped again, this lasting for nearly a year after the episode. Many people think back to the accident for years afterwards with gradually diminishing anxiety. Bursts of intense desperation can abruptly recur decades later. Some describe the episode as being almost depersonalized and dreamlike.

An American air force pilot who was injured on a training flight in 1958 described with detachment making an emergency landing and the fuel catching fire and seeing his clothes and harness burning as he struggled to get out of the plane. Twenty five years after this event, he recalls it but at a great psychological distance. Another description of a burn injury was written by Richard Hillary who was shot down in the Battle of Britain. He wrote:

I felt a terrific explosion which knocked the control stick from my hand. The whole machine quivered like a stricken animal. In a second, the cockpit was a mass of flames: instinctively, I reached up to open the hood. It would not move. I tore off my straps and managed to force it back; but this took time, and I dropped back into the seat and reached for the stick in an effort to turn the plane on it's back, the heat was so intense that I could feel myself going. I remember a second of sharp agony, remember thinking (so this is it!) and putting both hands to my eyes. Then I passed out. When I regained conscious-ness, I was free of the machine and falling rapidly. I saw that my left trouser leg was burned off and that I was going to fall into the sea . . . .

I felt faintly sick from the smell of burnt flesh. By closing my one eye, I could see my lips jutting out like motor tires . . . My hands were burnt and so judging from the pain of the sun was my face.

A few minutes later floating in the English Channel, he said:

I looked down at my hands and not seeing them realized that I had gone blind. So I was going to die. It came to me like that — I was going to die, and I was not afraid. Then realization came as a surprise. The manner of my approaching death appalled and horrified me but the actual vision of death left me unafraid; I felt only a profound curiosity and a sense of satisfaction that within a few minutes or a few hours, I was to learn the great answer.

This is a skillful and typical evocation of the altered consciousness of many people in burn situations. Hillary survived a long period in the hospital during his treatment and went out courageously in public with a mummified appearance.

Preoccupation with death is very much part of burn patients' concerns during the months in the hospital. At the time they are nearest death, they are not clear enough of mind to be occupied with it but during the months in the hospital, patients begin to think that they will endure an endless trial of being disfigured, misshapen, helpless, and unable to cope with their lives. They have an awareness that the very course of life itself has been altered and altered for the worst. No cliches about the sweetness of adversity make a serious impact amidst the agonies that confront the burned individual. There is a sense of being excluded from the mainstream of life. Some of the women survivors of Hiroshima felt 20 years after being scarred that they were no longer fully existing and were suffering "Death in Life" (Lifton, 1967).

After several months in the hospital when the patient begins to be more active, the downcast mood seems to lift. There is more energy to do things and there are more distractions. The isolation techniques are modified and the patient is usually out on a ward. He is able to talk to other people, to have visitors, and to talk more about what he will be doing. The immediate things that occupy him are stressful physical therapy activities—exercising his hands, starting to walk, immersion in hydrotherapy, trying to tighten up muscles that have atrophied through disuse, attempting to see that tendons that have been shifted are being used, and scooting around in a wheelchair to see other patients and try out social skills again. Some patients find this very frightening, that after having been regressed and passive for so long, they have to do things for themselves. They have been fed; they have been toileted; their bodies have been washed; and now more is expected of them. While this may produce only a passing tremor in most individuals, for a few patients it is so upsetting that they will not attempt to be active in any way. It causes them to battle with the physical therapists and to evade planning for return to work and home and can delay rehabilitation for months.

RELIGION

The burn units of most hospitals have chaplains available. Pastoral care training programs are developing in some institutions. However, pastoral counseling and the work of the chaplain is very much thrust aside by the functioning of medical technology of a burn centre and the specialization of human care services such as those of the psychiatrist and social worker. It is also true that clergymen often feel overwhelmed by technology and cannot function in these settings. They feel they have little to offer. It is also striking that in modern burn units, patients do not often call for religious help but instead are referred to mental health professionals or make relationships with the staff and talk to the nurses informally about their hopes and beliefs. One of the problems that many nurses report is patients asking them early on, "Will I live?" or "Why did this happen to me?" when the nurse is changing a dressing and not expecting serious discussion. Later, as the patients feel better, they ask, "What will I look like?" "Can I see a mirror?" Policies about whether patients should see themselves early vary. Some nurses will sneak in a mirror, some will insist that patients look at themselves. In most circumstances, there is a balance between the readiness of the patient and the directives of the staff about when they start focusing on personal appearance. The pastoral counselors who have been most successful with burn patients have generally taken on a clear social work rather than a religious role. This does not exclude some conventional members of the clergy who do their pastoral counseling jobs directly and well, nor the very religious patients whose faith sustains them. In times of catastrophe, intense belief of many kinds avails much. Psychiatrists in Shanghai (Zhangi Xia, personal communication, November 24, 1983) note that burn patients who managed their suffering and disfigurement best were "those who had a complete belief in Communism." Men who were absolutely driven to get back to their families also fared better.

Womach and White (1976) recounted how Womach's injury and burn disfigurement were made tolerable by his religious faith that "out of suffering came joy . . . God has shaped suffering into something beautiful." It is common for patients to have get well cards pasted on the walls all around them but a few burn patients will insist on having pictures of what they looked like before the accident put up as a steady reminder of what they once were. They derive some strength from knowing about this—seeing themselves as previously complete, attractive, and competent. Others are appalled and thrust into despair over what they have lost.

Wright (1960) has reported that for some people the experience of being handicapped leads them to feel more tolerant, more philosophical, and more accepting about life. Most clinical experience indicates that this is only an occasional occurrence and that bitterness, despair, and constriction of the personality are by far more common reactions to what has happened. When patients begin to face the return to home, community, and jobs, they confront these challenges as altered deviant individuals. Their metamorphosis is discernible. They are weaker, they frequently seem older, "facing it," is a grimly relevant term. Facial scars make them stand out and be scapegoated and also make it harder for them to express ordinary emotions. Their features may be frozen in their scars. Children and spouses report they have to "relearn" the expressions in the scarred patient's face. They are dependent on the hospital for years in terms of scheduling new procedures, having scars that tighten up released, having continuing cosmetic reconstructive surgery planned so that they have an umbilical cord to the hospital that is both clinically necessary and emotional. Where it has been said that for cancer patients there is the chronic fear and hazard of dying, for the burn patient leaving the hospital presents the hazard and tremendous challenge of having to live as fully as possible.

Mechanic (1974) wrote that to cope in such circumstances requires several components.

1. A person must have capabilities and skills to deal with the social and environmental demands to which he is exposed: coping capabilities.
2. A person must be motivated to meet the demands that become evident in the environment.
3. A person must have the emotional capacity to maintain a state of psychological equilibrium so that he can direct energies and skills to meeting external, as well as internal distress.

These are dealt with in an infinite variety of styles and circumstances. As burn patients go home, they often stay there for a long period of time.

Case 5

John, who returned to his job, described what he said to himself, "John, either you're going to hide in your house or you're getting out there and face the world." He had lost one hand and all the features of his face had been grossly altered with his hair burned off. He had a devoted wife and children and a number of supportive friends. In recounting this, he did not have any memory of what his wife described; that he had hidden in the house for 3 years in despair before doing anything in public. But then he went back to a clerical job and after 50 operations and 20 years remained employed and socially active. He maintained a style of quickly talking to strangers he met, "So that they can know that I'm human."

Case 6

Another patient, Gertrude, described in a television documentary (Marin & Moseley, 1982) about disfigurement, that for 7 years after she had been badly burned she simply existed in hiding and in the eighth year she began to go out and face the world and feel differently about it. She described herself as a phoenix who had risen from the ashes of her own life. She now goes out and has a varied, active life, but at the price of continuing effort, irritability, and some bitterness about society's reactions.

Many patients make resolves but they do not follow through on them. Many are very much like old people for whom the phrase, "burn out" is an unfortunate pun. Cowley in "The View From Eighty" (1976) says that when he sits in his chair he feels he is still the same energetic person he had been all his life but once he actually tries to get up and move around, he feels all the infirmities of age. The burn patient has often been changed in this way as well. Many feel devitalized. They speak of being weaker and of being exhausted by the chores of getting up, dressing, bearing all the weight of their scars, and having a limited range of motion.

Another large area that distinguishes them from cardiacs or people with cancer or many other nonvisible handicaps is that burn injuries so often are unsightly and society does not easily accept people who look frightening. Many burn patients feel they have been converted into *things*. As one patient stated it, "Am I no longer a man?" after his face had been very severely burned. A young woman, who had been a high school cheerleader in a small town said she had become sexless and also said she was a *thing* after being in a fire which disfigured her face, hands, and breasts.

Some patients become very assertive sexually. One 17-year-old California high school girl became aggressively sexual after facial and hand burn disfigurement from an auto accident in which her date was driving while drunk. She was very promiscuous, to the outrage of her Mormon parents, diverting from herself the dejected feelings she had about the deformation of her face and body, and counterphobically rushing at boys who might reject her. Most avoided her nervously.

For patients who go back to a stable life the outlook is better. If they have a family, they usually have the support that gives them a much better chance of making an adaptation. There may be all manner of problems within the family members in their own feelings about disfiguration but they will usually accept the patient and suppress most of their sadness. Siblings and spouses try to squelch their negative reactions. Sometimes patients utter cliches about how they feel they are more beautiful inside because of what has happened. Most are mute on this subject. The major difficulty that patients talk about is the way they look and the way they are treated. The young physicist who had been burned trying to rescue someone in a fire said that when he went for a job interview, the man interviewing him "couldn't wait to get out of the room" because of the way the patient looked. People turn aside, they look shocked, they make whispered remarks. The burn patient who is disfigured must permanently reserve energy and be on guard to deal with these social contingencies. This is very different from a serious cardiac or somebody with a nonvisible carcinoma who carries a grave burden but not one which will be abruptly and unexpectedly brought up by strangers in almost any public situation. For this, the burn patient has to be ready and has to have answers about what happened. He must be ready to respond, whether to joke or engage people's sympathy. Once the scarring and disfigurement is brought up in a conversation, reactions to it tend to inundate whatever else is going on. When people ask, "What are you?" all other issues fade.

Some burn patients have taken the position that they prefer to be asked what has happened and then will reply, it was a fire. Some of them say things like, "This is what happened to me. Ain't I gorgeous?" or attempt to set a tone of levity that they believe puts other people at ease. Some simply shrink away.

Giving-up and giving-in has been described as a way of explaining the background for some psychosomatic diseases. It fits the commonsense idea that a person's frame of mind relates to his propensity for illness or death. It is clear that discouragement, despair, humiliation, and grief are conducive to illness whereas contentment, happiness, hope, confidence, and success are usually associated with good health. However, for burn patients who feel helpless and hopeless, there is not necessarily an increase in psychosomatic disease but rather a decrease in successful adaptation to the altered life situation that they must live in. When they give up, they withdraw and can pull back from normal living altogether. What happens to them was described many years ago by Macgregor (1953) as *social death,* which she describes as the social withdrawal of disfigured people and the severance of their personal contacts. Such people become closet people. The number of suicides among them is not fully known, but anecdotal information clearly shows it to be significant.

Moos and Tsu (1977) ask what factors influence the overall appraisal of an illness, the perception of specific tasks and the initial choice of coping skills and subsequent changes in coping strategy? The relevant determinants fall into three categories: background and physical characteristics, illness related factors, and features of the physical and sociocultural environment. These are certainly realistic generalities, but they remain generalities. The personality qualities which enable a particular person to handle a catastrophic burn injury are difficult to elicit from a general backgound history. No illness is analogous to a burn in most peoples' lives so that a history of broken legs in football games or even hypochrondriasis and many visits to the doctor will not give a good prognostic indicator. Certainly, the observation that strong and vigorous personalities will do better is a reasonable starting point but it is difficult to make precise predictions because of the vast multitude of social and individual factors involved. A large number of burn patients simply disappear from medical care. They do not come back for follow up. As stated, we are not aware how many commit suicide or what percentage go into the closet. We are clearly aware that most of them are not visible in the general public so that a good assumption is that most facially burned, scarred individuals choose a life path that keeps them from public view. The experience of the burn itself is transformed into an experience of long hospitalization and medical care but then the patients cast themselves into an altered or handicapped life style in which they live not as chronically ill people but as deviant individuals who do not fit society's standards for functioning (Bernstein 1976, 1983).

Many people manage all of this and proceed with their lives after they leave medical care but the statistics remain unclear. How many succeed and how many succumb? The burned, disfigured person has been changed from an unremarkable looking individual into one whose appearance becomes an issue as soon as he enters a new situation. There is now a constant burden to make oneself acceptable to people who might be frightened. The burden is unfairly placed on the patient. Patients can flaunt their scars, but this makes many people avoid them. They can evade society on the "social death" route. Or they can pursue the normal ends of living, working, loving, and being productive, bearing the continuing burden that their injuries have produced.

REFERENCES

Allport, G. (1942). The use of personal documents in psychological science. *Social Science Research Council Bulletin 2.*

Bernstein, N. R. (1976). *Emotional Care of the Facially Burned and Disfigured.* Boston: Little, Brown and Company.

Bernstein, N. R. & Robson, M. C. (Eds.) (1983). *Comprehensive Approaches to the Burned Person.* New Hyde Park, New York: Medical Examination Publishing Company.

Cousins, N. (1981). *Human Options.* New York: Norton.

Cowley, M. (1976). *The View from Eighty.* New York: Penguin.

Hillary, Richard (1983). *The Last Enemy.* New York: St. Martin's.

Lifton, R. J. (1967). *Death in Life.* New York: Random House.

Macgregor, F. C. (Ed.). (1953). *Facial Deformities and Plastic Surgery: A Psychosocial study,* Springfield, IL: Thomas.

Marin, C., & Moseley, D. (1982). *Beauty Passed Away* [NBC Film Documentary]. Chicago.

Mechanic, D. (1974). Social structural and personal adaptation: Some neglected dimensions. In G. V. Coelho, D. A. Hamburg, & J. E. Adams (Eds.), *Coping and Adaptation.* New York: Basic Bks.

Moos, R. H., & Tsu, U. D. (1977). The crisis of physical illness: An overview. In R. H. Moos (Ed.), *Coping with Physical Illness.* New York: Plenum.

Mosely, L. (1962). *Faces From the Fire.* Englewood Cliffs, NS: Prentice-Hall.

Perry, S. (1983). The undermedication for pain: a psychoanalytic perspective. *Association for Psychoanalytic Medicine Bulletin, 22,* 77–93.

Schilder, P. (1950). *The Image and Appearance of the Human Body.* New York: International Universities.

Womach, M. V., & White, M. L. (1976). *Tested by Fire.* Old Tappan, Fleming, H. Revell.

Wright, B. (1960). *Physical Disability: A Psychological Approach.* New York: Harper & Row.

Bypass Surgery for Superobesity: The Patient's Experience

PIETRO CASTELNUOVO-TEDESCO, M.D.

Obesity is a remarkably complex disorder in which many factors (genetic, anatomic, endocrine, biochemical, neuroregulatory, and nutritional as well as psychologic, social, and cultural) play variable roles. Because of its complexity and our inability to control satisfactorily any of the etiologic factors, many forms of treatment have been tried: all leave much to be desired and have presented a range of problems (Bray and Benfield, 1977; Van Itallie, 1980). The disparate methods used in the quest for a solution to this difficult condition have included diets, starvation, anorectic drugs, exercise, psychotherapeutic approaches of various sorts, membership in weight reduction groups, and surgical interventions.

Conservative therapeutic measures have proven both unreliable and unsatisfactory methods of achieving weight control. It is not surprising, therefore, that in recent years more radical approaches have been considered for cases of extreme obesity, commonly termed superobesity or morbid obesity (Van Itallie, 1980). Surgical treatment, in fact, has come into common use for this disorder—one might be tempted to call it a popular treatment, even though it remains an issue of some controversy.

The basic operations for the control of superobesity are two, jejuno-ileal bypass and gastric bypass, although several variants of each have been developed. Jejuno-ileal bypass is approximately 25 years old and has been used in thousands of patients, both in this country and abroad (DeWind & Payne, 1976; Payne, DeWind, & Commons, 1963; Scott, Shull et al., 1977). Gastric bypass, a more recent operation, has been available for over 10 years and has received steadily increasing attention and acceptance (Gomez, 1980; Mason & Ito, 1969; Mason, Printen, Blommers et al., 1980). These operations are reserved for persons whose weight is at least twice their ideal weight or who weigh more than 250–300 pounds (Bray & Benfield, 1977; Faloon, 1977; Scott et al., 1977).

In short, over the past 2 decades these procedures have been used extensively and, as a result, much has been learned about the experience of the average patient who undergoes this form of treatment (as far back as July 1976, a review of the literature on intestinal bypass alone counted 226 articles [Phillips, 1978] and much has been added on both forms of bypass since then). A discussion of the topic requires that some attention be given to the psychological characteristics of superobese patients, to the nature of the procedures that have been used, and finally to patients' reports and to the results that have been observed. The sections that follow will address these issues.

PSYCHOLOGICAL CHARACTERISTICS OF SUPEROBESE PATIENTS

There is uncertainty in the literature about the psychological characteristics of obese patients and over the years the topic has brought forth a variety of views. The situation is similar with regard to superobesity. Briefly, the older literature, dating back to the 1930s, 1940s, and early 1950s, was characterized by a psychoanalytic orientation and by tendency to see obese patients as suffering from pronounced personality disturbances (Bychowski, 1950; Hamburger, 1951; Hecht, 1955; Rascovsky, deRascovsky, and Schlossberg, 1950; Richardson, 1946; Wulff, 1932). Descriptions were in terms of analytic concepts of orality; oral trends resulted from fixation at that level or from regression after failure to master the oedipal situation. In this context, emphasis was given to patients' dependency, emotional liability, insatiableness, and proneness to depression. Indeed, at that time the view of obesity as a depressive equivalent was widely accepted as a clinical truism.

The orientation of the literature changed during the late 1950s, 1960s and early 1970s mainly as a result of the contributions of Stunkard (1959; and Stunkard & McLaren-Hume, 1959; Stunkard & Mendelson, 1961; Weinberg, Mendelson, & Stunkard, 1961; Mendelson, Weinberg, & Stunkard, 1961) and Bruch (1957, 1973). Stunkard, in particular, brought a needed corrective to the overly definitive and fairly restrictive formulations typical of that time. He questioned much that had been taken for granted, noting that "it has not even been possible to define psychological characteristics of obese persons which will consistently distinguish them from nonobese persons" (Stunkard, 1959). He also concluded that they cannot be distinguished from an unselected general population in terms of demonstrable psychopathology (Weinberg et al., 1961). Stunkard's views, however, while adding an important note of rigor and objectivity, possibly may have gone too far in the direction of skepticism. Bruch, a psychoanalyst, offered in her extensive writings a comprehensive dynamic understanding of the obese. Yet, by emphasizing the great diversity of their clinical manifestations and adaptive performances (Bruch, 1973, p. 132), she also has tended, like Stunkard, to counter the earlier view of the obese that stressed the uniformity of their characteristics.

In the last decade or so relatively few studies have addressed the psychological characteristics of obese or superobese patients. This occurred, in no small part, because during this period research interest has been directed mainly at issues deemed more accessible to objective assessment (e.g., the types of obesity [Mendelson et al., 1961], the eating patterns of the obese [Stunkard, 1959], the circumstances that favor overeating [Rodin, 1976; Stunkard, Grace, Wolff, 1955], and the emotional complications of weight reduction [Bruch, 1952; Kollar, Atkinson and Albin 1969; Stunkard, 1957]).

Recent research on the psychological characteristics of the superobese has been carried out mainly in conjunction with studies of these patients' response to intestinal bypass surgery. These studies have not provided a fully consistent or comprehensive view of obese patients. A factor to be noted is that patients who receive bypass surgery basically are self-selected and may not be truly representative of the larger pool of superobese persons. Also, the number of patients studied psychiatrically in this context has not been large. Finally, as Charles, Blumberg, Mozello et al., (in press) have suggested, there may be psychological differences not only between the obese and the superobese, but also between the superobese and the "super-super" obese (i.e., those whose weight is more than 200 pounds above their ideal weight). In short, more extensive and systematic investigations are needed; specifically, it would be helpful to compare the psychological characteristics of persons at various levels of obesity. Nonetheless, available studies permit at least some tentative generalizations.

A disturbance of the body image is a cardinal feature of the obese and superobese. This, in fact, is the one characteristic about which there is a consensus in the literature (Stunkard & Mendelson [1961] consider it, together with overeating, the *only* form of neurotic behavior specifically related to obesity). Central to the body image disturbance is an overwhelming preoccupation with one's obesity, a sense that one's body is loathsome and grotesque and likely to be viewed by others with horror and contempt (Stunkard & Mendelson, 1961). The body image disturbance is not a uniform occurrence and may present with varying intensity. It is associated especially with early onset of obesity, with disturbed family relationships in childhood and with negative parental view of one's obesity; some persons with adult onset obesity may be free of it (Stunkard & Burt, 1967; Stunkard & Mendelson, 1961).

A most important issue pertains to the degree and kind of emotional pathology found in these patients. From a study of superobese women, Castelnuovo-Tedesco and Schiebel (1975, 1976) have suggested that the majority are surprisingly free of extreme psychopathology. In particular, psychosis or crippling neurosis rarely seem to occur in this group. This finding often evokes disbelief in those who have not had direct contact with these patients. Many are inclined to assume (as we also did initially) that persons with massive distortions of the body shape, a serious and obvious handicap to adaptation, inevitably must show severe psychopathology. Yet, this has proven not to be the case, a finding which other investigators have confirmed (Atkinson & Ringuette, 1967; Halmi, Long, Stunkard et al., 1980; Holland, Masling, & Copley, 1970; Hutzler, Keen, Molinari et al., 1981; Leon, Eckert, Teed et al., 1979; Reivich, Ruiz, & Lapi, 1966; Swanson & Dinello, 1970; Webb, Phares, Abram et al., 1976; Wise & Fernandez, 1979). What one finds in studying these patients, is the presence, generally, of a mild to moderate personality disturbance in which passive-dependent and passive-aggressive traits predominate (Atkinson & Ringuette, 1967; Castelnuovo-Tedesco & Schiebel, 1975, 1976; Hutzler et al., 1981; Reivich et al., 1966; Swanson & Dinello, 1970; Webb et al., 1976). Some (Hutzler et al., 1981) specifically mention poor impulse control. Mild to moderate depression, frequently disguised by a facade of jolliness, is common among

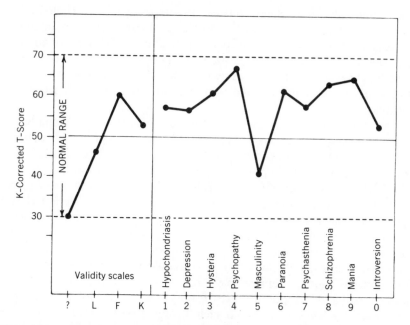

Figure 11.1.   Average preoperative MMPI profile. *Source:* Castelnuovo-Tedesco, P. & Schiebel, D. (1975). Copyright 1975, Int. Journal of Psychiatry in Medicine. Reprinted by permission.

the superobese, but severe and incapacitating depressive trends are seldom seen (Reivich et al., 1966). Figure 11.1 shows the average MMPI profile of a group of 12 superobese women; it is within normal limits (Castelnuovo-Tedesco & Schiebel, 1975). Webb et al. (1976), from their study of 70 patients, similarly concluded that "severe psychological problems are rare, but mild emotional immaturity is frequent, indeed modal." Wise & Fernandez (1979) also found a low level of psychopathology. Of 24 patients, only 2 had a diagnosable disturbance (in both cases a secondary affective disorder by research criteria). They add "As a group they presented as pleasant, appropriate individuals." Holland et al. (1970) compared groups of normal-weight, obese and superobese, white, lower class women and found no significant differences as to psychopathology. These authors also emphasized the contribution of social class membership in determining the "acceptability" of obesity and therefore the likelihood that it will be associated with psychopathology. Obesity appears much more acceptable in the lower than the upper social classes. Others (Meyer & Tuchelt-Gallwiz, 1963) have made similar points. Indirect evidence that most superobese possess at least a fair degree of psychological health is to be found in the experience with bypass operations. It is significant that these procedures have been accomplished in large numbers for 25 years, usually with little or no psychiatric screening or follow-up, yet with very few serious psychiatric complications.

The question of psychiatric diagnosis and degree of psychopathology among the superobese has been complicated, rather than simplified, by the introduction of The Diagnostic and Statistical Manual III(DSM III). Two studies (Charles et al., in press; Halmi, Long et al., 1980) so far have used DSM III criteria, with differing results. Halmi, Long et al. (1980), who studied 80 patients, found that the lifetime prevalence of Axis I clinical psychiatric diagnoses was 47.5 percent, with depressive disorders occurring in 28.7 percent of the total sample. They report that this compares with a rate of depressive disorder of 24.7 percent in the general population. By contrast, Charles et al. (in press), who studied 15 patients, found that the prevalence of lifetime depressive disorder was 53 percent, while 47 percent had a personality disorder on Axis II; only one person had no diagnosable mental illness. They suggest that such divergent results occur because this population is not homogeneous. This is likely, but may not be the main issue. Relevant also may be some characteristics of DSM III. Despite the presence of Axis V ("highest level of functioning in the past year"), DSM III, by its emphasis on "counting symptoms," has difficulty giving weight to the patient's personality strengths. This may do a disservice to many patients in the psychoneurotic and borderline range. In addition to their psychopathology, they may demonstrate significant assets and resources that are difficult to include in the assessment. For these reasons, the superobese may appear "sicker" when diagnosed by DSM III criteria; many may be labeled as having an "affective disorder" when, from another point of view, they might be seen as having a personality disorder, tinged with depression.

Another important finding from studies of the superobese is the frequent occurrence of family instability in the early experience of these patients (Castelnuovo-Tedesco & Schiebel, 1975). Parental separation or divorce is a common childhood event. For a variety of reasons, the patient's mother typically has not provided consistent care, interest, and understanding, and the patient has been left, often rather prematurely, to depend on his or her own resources. In this setting, food often serves as a readily available and dependable source of support, satisfaction, and consolation. Even in poor families, food is available in large quantities and comes to be regarded as a ready means of providing for oneself without having to depend on others. Fink, Gottesfeld, and Glickman (1962) found that 55 percent of their 31 superobese patients had experienced separation from one or both parents early in childhood; conflict with, and poor care by, parents had been a frequent occurrence. Early parental loss, separation from parents or family instability, was a common finding in other reports as well (Atkinson & Ringuette, 1967; Reivich et al., 1966).

Yet another significant finding is these patients' attitude toward food which, superficially at least, is both positive and unambivalent (Castelnuovo-Tedesco & Schiebel, 1975). They regard all food with joy and pleasure and are able to eat it in large quantities without suffering any of the usual distress that many normally experience if they overeat. This capacity to eat large amounts of food without ill effect certainly contributes to the obese person's difficulty controlling his or her intake and recognizing how much food is actually ingested. In other words, these patients are inclined to under-estimate how much they eat and commonly resort to rationalization and denial to explain their obesity. For example, they will say that it is due to some obscure metabolic disturbance or to eating the wrong foods. It is difficult for them to acknowledge that they eat excessively or even that they eat more than most people do.

Obesity, which influences the body image so much, also shapes these patients' identity (Castelnuovo-Tedesco & Schiebel, 1975). They think of themselves, above all, as people who are *fat* and this awareness is seldom absent from their consciousness. Stunkard and Mendelson (1967) call it their "overriding concern." They are reminded of this by aspects of their physical environment (e.g., by difficulty finding ready-made clothes or fitting into ordinary chairs or car seats) or by the attention of others. They dislike their obesity intensely and they carefully avoid mirrors, scales, and any situation that might confirm this perception. For example, they typically are most unwilling to be seen in a bathing suit, and even in the context of marriage or other intimate relationship they avoid undressing before their spouse or partner (Castelnuovo-Tedesco & Schiebel, 1975).

Also, they often show a distinct lack of curiosity and interest in their own psychological functioning as well as a rather limited capacity for introspection (Castelnuovo-Tedesco & Schiebel, 1975). This was well demonstrated when 12 superobese women, who were candidates for jejuno-ileal bypass, were offered the opportunity to be seen in regular once-a-week psychotherapy without charge. None of the women availed herself of this offer, preferring instead to be seen in monthly follow-up visits or to call for a special appoint-ment if one experienced some acute difficulty (Castelnuovo-Tedesco &

Schiebel, 1975). It became clear that, except in emergencies, these patients prefer to handle their own affairs without resorting to outside help; they do not like to consider themselves psychiatric patients or to address personal issues of long standing. However, there was no lack of capacity or interest in forming a relationship. Despite their unwillingness to participate in regularly scheduled formal psychotherapy, most patients maintained a friendly contact with the psychiatrist and seemed pleased when he called them to arrange for monthly follow-up interviews. Similarly, in a study of obese men by Mendelson et al. (1961), approximately half of the group did not accept the offer of weekly psychotherapy. Werkman and Greenberg (1967) found that obese adolescent girls attempted to present themselves as "hypernormal" and were defensive about revealing any psychological problems. Reivich et al. (1966) described their group of 33 superobese patients as "essentially unaware of emotional problems" and as "tenuously motivated" for psychotherapy. "Immaturity and lack of psychological sophistication" were characteristic of the female superobese patients of Hutzler et al. (1981).

Before concluding this section, it must be repeated that, in working with obese and superobese patients, one often notes the prominence of passive-aggressive traits, notably stubbornness and defiance (Castelnuovo-Tedesco and Schiebel, 1975). Similar observations have been made by Bruch (1952), Reivich, Ruiz et al. (1966), Swanson & Dinello (1970), Fink et al. (1962), Kollar and Atkinson (1966). Dependency needs in many cases are not impressively manifest; striking rather is the struggle *against* dependency, which expresses itself in significant needs for independence and autonomy (Castelnuovo-Tedesco & Schiebel, 1975). Although desirous of help and support, these patients are inclined to convey their mistrust of others as well as their resentment that others do not help more readily. Many have learned from early experience that, despite their sense of inadequacy, it is safer to look after oneself. Thus, they are wary of entangling relationships. These characteristics help to explain, if only partially, why the obese traditionally have been regarded as "difficult" patients, why typically they are refractory to treatment programs based on adherence to diet, and why they tend to be not very psychologically minded.

In summary, although the diagnostic or psychodynamic characteristics just mentioned cannot be used to differentiate this group from patients with other psychosomatic disorders, one is impressed nonetheless by a certain consistency, indeed by considerable repetitiveness, in the material from case to case. This brings to mind a comment by Engel (1955) about ulcerative colitis. He noted that although it would be misleading to consider certain personality traits as specifically identified with that disease, "given the diagnosis of ulcerative colitis, the possibility of describing the major character traits of the patient without even seeing him is excellent." Engel's observation seems applicable also to superobesity.

SURGICAL TREATMENT OF SUPEROBESITY

The goal of surgical treatment is to reduce permanently either the intake or the absorption of food (Hallberg, 1980). Most procedures combine both of these principles. Gastric bypass acts primarily by reducing intake, although absorption also is reduced in a "true" gastric bypass. Jaw wiring, a relatively simple procedure, acts solely by reducing food intake. Jejuno-ileal bypass originally was thought to act primarily by reducing food absorption (Payne et al., 1963); recent evidence, however, suggests that reduced intake is more important than what once was believed (Sclafani, 1981).

Intestinal bypass surgery was introduced clinically in the late 1950s by Payne and DeWind (Payne et al., 1963) of Los Angeles. They first tried a jejuno-colic anastomosis but soon discarded it because of serious side effects; their next operation was a jejuno-ileal anastomosis which has remained through the years the basic intestinal bypass procedure. Several variants of this operation have been tried. Currently three forms are most commonly employed: Payne and DeWind's original "14 + 4" (i.e., 14 inches of jejunum anastomosed end to side to 4 inches of ileum) and Scott's "12 + 8" or "12 + 6" (i.e., 12 inches of jejunum anastomosed to 8 or 6 inches of ileum, end to end) (DeWind & Payne, 1976; Payne et al., 1963; Scott et al., 1977). The Payne and the Scott procedures are in common use today and all appear to be about equally popular (Gaspar et al., 1976).

The term "gastric bypass" refers to several alternative procedures that may be used to reduce the functional gastric cavity and thus also food intake. The operation creates an antral pouch of approximately 50 cc capacity with an exit stoma of approximately 12 mm in diameter. This can be accomplished either by gastric partition or by gastroplasty ("stapling") (Gomez, 1980; Mason et al., 1980). Gastric partition or gastroplasty may also be combined with a gastroenteric anastomosis by connecting the small gastric pouch with a loop of jejunum; in such cases one may properly speak of a true gastric bypass.

In the discussion to follow, bear in mind that both intestinal and gastric bypass are major surgical interventions with significant risks of morbidity and mortality. The mortality for jejuno-ileal bypass is approximately 3 to 4 percent at major medical centers, although in a few reports it has been over 10 percent. Morbidity includes all the somatic complications that may follow any major abdominal procedure as well as others which are characteristic of intestinal bypass surgery (Bray & Benfield, 1977; Pi-Sunyer, 1976; Scott et al., 1977).These commonly include diarrhea, electrolyte disturbances, hypoproteinemia, as well as involvement of the liver, kidneys, and joints. There may also be manifestations of obstruction in the defunctionalized bowel (so-called "bypass enteritis"). Over 50 percent of patients suffer some complications (Bray & Benfield, 1977). These may be very serious and may require reoperation to reestablish normal intestinal continuity; reversal of the bypass may be essential to save the patient's life. A point of some importance is the timing of the complications after jejuno-ileal bypass. Briefly, the first 3 years after the operation, which is the period of rapid weight loss, is the time when serious complications are most likely to occur. After the first 3 years, the patient's condition tends to stabilize both in terms of weight and of relative freedom from serious complications. On the other hand, late serious complications are not totally excluded and, in particular, uropathies and arthropathies may occur well after the third year (Pi-Sunyer, 1976; Scott et al., 1977).

Gastric bypass has different complications from jejuno-ileal bypass and is generally regarded as a safer operation. Mortality is in the range of .5 to 3 percent (Buchwald, 1980; Gomez, 1980; Mason et al., 1978; 1980). The principal difficulties are limited to the very early postoperative period; also, the serious metabolic abnormalities that may follow intestinal bypass do not occur after gastric bypass. More specifically, there are no electrolyte, liver, kidney, gall bladder, or joint problems. There is also no abdominal distension or diarrhea. On the other hand, other problems may occur that are characteristic of gastric bypass. These include vomiting, rupture of the suture line, and stretching of the gastric pouch. The last two make the operation ineffective, so that ultimately reoperation becomes necessary. Leakage of the gastroenteric anastomosis may result in peritonitis, intraabdominal or subphrenic abscesses (Buckwalter & Herbst, 1980). There may also be stomal ulceration or dumping syndrome. Prolonged vomiting may result in avitaminosis and malnutrition and may present with a peripheral neuritis or a mild dementia. In other words, although gastric bypass generally is considered safer than intestinal bypass, it is not entirely free of difficulties and occasionally these are serious.

Finally, a brief account will be given of jaw wiring. Its principal asset is that it does not involve a major surgical procedure and carries no particular risk. Therefore, it may be employed to treat mild as well as severe cases of obesity. It is appropriate for patients who are 30 to 50 pounds overweight as well as for those who weigh over 300 pounds (Castelnuovo-Tedesco, Buchanan, & Hall, 1980; Kark, 1980).

Jaw wiring has been available for some time, but it has been used mainly by dentists and has not yet received extensive study. Jaw wiring (temporo-mandibular fixation) involves placing small buttons on the premolars and then wiring these buttons together to keep the jaws shut. The patient is given an 800 calorie liquid diet, and, if adhered to, weight loss follows in a very dependable way (Castelnuovo-Tedesco et al., 1980; Kark, 1980). Unfortunately, the problem with jaw wiring is that patient compliance generally is poor. Interestingly, the complications of jaw wiring result from certain psychological aspects of the procedure. The procedure itself is not painful nor is the day-to-day wearing of the wires. Also, they do not interfere with speech. Patients, however, find the wires confining and unpleasant over long periods. Paradoxically, most patients in the beginning respond to jaw wiring with enthusiasm. They are pleased that they are finally losing weight after many years of fruitless efforts, and they enjoy the compliments that they receive from relatives and friends. However, after the initial enthusiastic response, patients begin to feel restricted by the wires and ultimately end up resenting them. Jaw wiring appears to mobilize these patients' not inconsiderable passive-aggressiveness with the result that sooner or later most "cheat" on their diet (Castelnuovo-Tedesco et al., 1980). As a consequence, they stop losing weight or actually regain some of the weight they have lost. This in turn leads to discouragement and frustration. For some, the restriction imposed by jaw wiring is so unacceptable, that they find a variety of excuses for clipping their wires.

Jaw wiring initially appeals both to patients and physicians because it seems easy and appears to demand very little from the patient, but this is not so. On the contrary, patients need to collaborate actively with the program; if they are unable to do so, the treatment will fail. As might be expected, those who respond best to jaw wiring are the more mature, well integrated and motivated patients. Jaw wiring is an example of a treatment that works well as long as there is good compliance; regrettably, the psychological aspects of the procedure markedly reduce its effectiveness (Castelnuovo-Tedesco et al., 1980). Nonetheless, jaw wiring may have value in the treatment of some superobese patients who, because of coexisting medical problems, are not candidates for bypass treatment (Garrow, 1980).

PATIENTS' EXPERIENCE OF SURGERY FOR SUPEROBESITY

In this section an attempt will be made to review the patient's course after the different forms of surgery for superobesity. Emphasis will be given to the patient's subjective experience. As noted earlier, however, these patients are not particularly prone to introspection or to communicating their introspections, so that the substance of their experience often has to be gauged by observation and inference.

Weight Loss

A critical aspect of the patient's experience after successful bypass surgery concerns the weight loss which occurs dramatically during the first postoperative year. Following intestinal bypass, most patients lose approximately 8 to 15 pounds per month. After the first critical year the weight loss gradually slows down, and after 2 or 3 years the weight generally stabilizes at between 150 and 200 pounds. Although this is seen by the patient as a great improvement, it is still considerably above the patient's "ideal" weight (Bray & Benfield, 1977; Castelnuovo-Tedesco & Schiebel, 1976). The average total weight loss is somewhere between 100 and 150 pounds. After the weight has stabilized, it remains approximately at this level for 10 years or more, although 2 to 3 years after surgery a modest weight gain may occur because the intestine is inclined to stretch and the absorbing mucosa hypertrophies. The period of active weight loss may be associated with a variety of physical symptoms and may be experienced by the patient as stressful, even though the manifestations of stress may be partially obscured by the patient's joyous satisfaction with the weight loss. The latter is seen as a major personal achievement; it also serves as an inducement to accept the physical discomforts that may accompany the procedure. Particularly in the first few weeks, patients may feel euphoric; they convey a sense of pleasurable excitement and often say that they "can't wait" to get down to a normal weight. Looking for trimmer clothes, feeling more "alive" and able to undertake physical activity, responding to the compliments and admiring comments from friends and relatives, create an atmosphere which the patient finds encouraging and narcissistically gratifying.

There are reports in the literature that psychological distress may be intensified if the weight loss is very rapid (Abram, Meixel, Webb et al., 1976; Crisp, Kalucy, Pilkington et al., 1977; Neill and Marshall, 1976). This, however is not well established. Indeed, there is evidence that the psychological distress may be related to concurrent medical problems rather than to the rapid weight loss, per se (Castelnuovo-Tedesco & Schiebel, 1976). At this stage, severe fatigue, weakness, nausea, and lack of appetite are not uncommon manifestations of electrolyte abnormalities or hepatic involvement. It is also well established that those who do not lose an adequate amount of weight, typically respond with frank unhappiness and disappointment.

Usually these patients seek reoperation to revise the bypass, so as to obtain, finally, the sought-after weight loss (Castelnuovo-Tedesco & Schiebel, 1976; Wise, 1976).

With regard to weight loss, the experience after gastric bypass is very similar to that after jejuno-ileal bypass. The principal difference is that after gastric bypass the weight loss proceeds somewhat more slowly and is slightly less (approximately 75 pounds) than after jejuno-ileal bypass (Mason et al., 1978; Scott, 1982).

After jaw wiring, the average weight loss is variable and depends on the patient's level of compliance with the program (Castelnuovo-Tedesco et al., 1980). Initially there is usually a fairly prompt weight loss which the patient finds gratifying. In the first month, patients lose an average of about 20 pounds. Total weight loss may reach as high as 30 or more pounds. Sooner or later, however, problems arise as resentment sets in at the restriction imposed by the wires. As previously mentioned, this leads to "cheating" on the diet, to regaining of weight, and to further discouragement and disappointment with the program.

Appetite and Food Intake

After jejuno-ileal bypass, weight loss occurs because there is reduction both of food intake and food absorption (Bray & Benfield, 1977; Castelnuovo-Tedesco & Schiebel, 1976; Sclafani 1981). During the first postoperative year, desire for food decreases noticeably and patients report that they eat less and less often than they did before surgery. Snacking and binge eating, which had been a prominent part of the preoperative eating pattern, decrease markedly or may be given up altogether. Patients also say that they now only eat one or two meals per day and that occasionally they even "forget" to eat for a whole day. They also tend to eat more in the morning and less at night (Bray, Dahms, Atkinson et al., 1980). The reasons for these changes in appetite and eating pattern have not been fully clarified, but an important factor is an aversive conditioning which occurs spontaneously after the operation and which serves to monitor and regulate food intake (Castelnuovo-Tedesco & Schiebel, 1976; Castelnuovo-Tedesco, 1980). More specifically, food intake promptly results in diarrhea, abdominal cramping, and flatus which are highly uncomfortable and interfere with further eating (patients typically try not to eat unless they are in a setting with ready access to a toilet). After surgery, patients become aware for the first time of a variety of new sensations originating from the gastrointestinal tract. Some patients can identify the passage of food through the intestine; it feels like it's "falling down a chute." These experiences contribute to a phenomenon of aversive conditioning and highlight an important characteristic of superobese patients: They may be said to possess truly "superior" gastrointestinal tracts. Before bypass surgery these patients had been remarkably free of ordinary digestive complaints. After bypass surgery they discover, for the first time, that uncomfortable gastrointestinal sensations can occur.

After jejuno-ileal bypass, patients report various changes in their taste preferences. Generally, sweets are less appealing. Subjective preference for a 40 percent sucrose solution is significantly lower than before surgery, although preference for 2.5, 5, or 10 percent solutions is not affected (Bray & Benfield, 1977; Bray et al., 1980). Thus, a patient who had eaten 1 pound of chocolate daily prior to intestinal bypass, had no candy for over 6 months after the operation (Rodin, 1980). Also, roughage, fried or spicy foods, tend to be avoided because they are irritating to the bowel and stimulate diarrhea (Castelnuovo-Tedesco & Schiebel, 1976; Castelnuovo-Tedesco 1980). Soft drinks are also avoided postoperatively, probably because of the high sugar content, while preoperatively they frequently had been used very liberally. Preference for sour (citric acid), salty, or bitter (quinine) tastes is virtually unchanged after surgery (Rodin, 1980). On the other hand, some patients report a craving or special liking for foods, such as fruits and vegetables, which often had not been a significant part of their preoperative diet (Castelnuovo-Tedesco & Schiebel, 1976). Postoperatively, as after dieting, there is no change in responsiveness to environmental stimuli (i.e., persons who are highly responsive remain vulnerable to the influence of salient and palatable food cues [Rodin, 1980]).

Usually after the first postoperative year (i.e., after gastrointestinal symptoms have subsided somewhat), food intake is likely to increase again so that after the third year it approximates once more the preoperative pattern (Castelnuovo-Tedesco & Schiebel, 1976). After several years, many patients again eat as much or nearly as much as they had preoperatively. We do not have, however, detailed studies of the late postoperative eating patterns. In a study of 8 patients, Bray, Zachary, Dahms et al. (1978) found that, prior to intestinal bypass, the daily caloric intake was nearly 7000 kcal. During the first 6 months after surgery, it dropped to less than 2000 kcal. It then rose to 3000 kcal after 1 year, to 4000 kcal after 2 years, and to approximately 5000 kcal after 3 years.

After gastric bypass, in order for the operation to be successful, the patient must promptly change his or her eating habits (Mason et al., 1978, 1980). Because the size of the functional stomach has been markedly reduced, the patient must learn at once to eat only small amounts with each meal. To accomplish this, surgeons generally give patients special instructions, before and immediately after the operation, on the importance of accommodating to the new gastric capacity (Gomez, 1980; Halverson, Zuckerman, Koehler et al., 1981). The smallness of the gastric pouch helps to reduce the appetite; it takes less food for the patient to achieve a comfortable sense of fullness. Most patients adapt to these changes without too much trouble and weight loss follows as expected. On the other hand, if the patient is unable to curb intake, vomiting is likely to result, followed by tearing of the suture lines and stretching of the gastric pouch. The latter outcome should be suspected if the patient does not show the anticipated steady weight loss. In short, the success of gastric bypass is conditional on the patient's capacity to cooperate; a true change in the patient's eating habits must take place. If not able to cooperate, the patient can "override" the procedure, either by eating too much at any one time (and stretching the gastric pouch), or by eating too frequently (thereby maintaining a high caloric intake) (Mason et al., 1978; Buchwald, 1980). According to Halmi, Mason, & Falk et al. (1981), thoughts about food and eating were much less frequent after gastric bypass than before. Patients also said that postoperatively they were more conscious of what they were eating and felt hungry much less often. In general, they said they enjoyed food to the same degree postoperatively as before. Patients also reported that they ate less often between meals, more slowly, drank liquids more often and found it easier to stop eating. The most significant reduction in food intake occurred in the calorically dense high carbohydrate foods, possibly because these tend to induce a dumping syndrome. Statistically significant decreases have been reported for all foods except fish, chicken, shell fish, vegetables, and alcoholic beverages. Decreased use of beef, pork, lamb, bread and cereals, butter and other fats, spicy foods, and sweets is especially marked (Harris & Green, 1982).

After jaw wiring, the patient must accept an 800 calorie liquid diet (Castelnuovo-Tedesco et al., 1980). This presents a considerable problem. Although patients do not complain of hunger or weakness, liquid low calorie diets tend to be monotonous and unsatisfying and soon contribute to the patient's irritability and to poor compliance which ultimately results in failure of the procedure. Efforts by the physician to improve compliance through encouragement and praise in most cases prove to be of limited practical value.

Postoperative Changes in Body Image

Disturbances of the body image are best considered in terms of its two components, the perceptual-cognitive and the affective. Unfortunately, however, this distinction has not been consistently observed in the literature.

The first component refers to the cognitive estimate of one's body size and shape, the second to the emotional response to one's physical characteristics as variously pleasing or unattractive.

A study by Schiebel and Castelnuovo-Tedesco (1978) investigated changes in patients' cognitive perception of their body size using a draw-a-person test. Patients were asked to draw a sketch of an "average person" and then a "self-sketch." These drawings were obtained prior to surgery and also 1 week, 3 months, and 1 year after surgery. Each patient's self-sketch and drawing of an "average person" were measured for maximal abdominal width and the results were converted into a ratio of self versus average size. This ratio then was compared in each case and at each point in time with the ratio of the patient's actual weight divided by the patient's expected weight (obtained from actuarial tables adjusted for height and age). The results (see Figure 11.2) show that superobese women had no difficulty assessing with reasonable accuracy their initial obesity and the gradual change in body size during the year that followed surgery. At the same time, a slight tendency was noted for patients to overestimate the weight loss actually achieved immediately after surgery; this was considered a "placebo" effect of the operation. There was also a similarly slight tendency for patients to over-estimate the weight loss achieved by the end of the first postoperative year. overall, patients were able to assess with reasonable accuracy the progressive changes in their body size. In other words, the perceptual-cognitive component of the body image seems essentially realistic and adapts promptly to

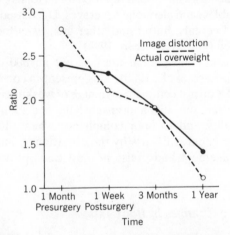

Figure 11.2. Comparison of ratios of average body image distortion to average normative overweight (N = 10). *Source:* Castelnuovo-Tedesco, P. & Schiebel, D. (1976). Copyright 1976, the American Psychiatric Association. Reprinted by permission.

the marked weight loss. On the other hand, the affective component of the body image appears to change much more slowly (Schiebel & Castelnuovo-Tedesco, 1978). It was studied by means of a sentence completion test (sample stems: "mirrors", "when I am naked", "handsome men"). Although the patients were pleased with their weight loss, 1 to 2 years after surgery they still retained distinctly dysphoric feelings about their bodies, which they continued to consider unattractive. In a similar vein, Stunkard and Burt (1967) have concluded that "the body image disturbances of obese persons are primarily affective rather than cognitive." Body size estimation, according to Leon et al. (1979), "showed a realistic adjustment with weight loss." Other investigators (Kalucy, Solow, Hartman, 1975), instead, have reported a lag in the response of the body image to the perception of weight loss. This lack of agreement probably is the result of differences in methodology and differences in distinguishing the perceptual-cognitive from the affective component of the body image. Ten or more years after the procedure, patients still retain dysphoric feelings about their appearance (Castelnuovo-Tedesco, Weinberg, Buchanan, 1982). One must note parenthetically that this dysphoria is not simply a consequence of persistent body image distortion. Schiebel and Castelnuovo-Tedesco (1978) said:

> Bypass surgery does not, automatically, bring physical attractiveness. In fact, as weight is lost, patients' skin tends to become pendulous and flabby and this is more distressing to some than their original appearance when their bodies were obese but firm. Often these patients become insistent on receiving plastic surgery to tighten loose skin and consider their treatment incomplete until this has been accomplished. In other words, after surgery a new reality factor is introduced and this probably also has bearing on why patients' feelings about their attractiveness do not show more significant change.

The previously mentioned studies were conducted with patients who received jejuno-ileal bypass. Less is known about patients who have received gastric bypass. The results, however, should not prove different, inasmuch as the distinguishing feature of each operation is the method by which weight loss is obtained rather than its outcome. Halmi, Stunkard, and Mason (1980), for example, found a marked decrease in body image disparagement and in mirror avoidance after gastric bypass, similar to their earlier findings after intestinal bypass.

Following jaw wiring, no significant changes have been noted in the body image, the average weight loss generally being too small to perceptibly influence this variable (Castelnuovo-Tedesco et al., 1980). Insofar as weight loss is achieved, patients are consistently pleased with this, but it does not alter significantly patients' impression that their bodies are unattractive; this, in turn, contributes to their ultimate dissatisfaction with the procedure.

Postoperative Adaptive Responses and Personal Adjustment

Before discussing patients' adaptive responses to bypass procedures, a comment is called for about the timing of the operation. Prior to the decision to undergo bypass surgery, most patients have experienced a period of heightened stress, as measured by the frequency of stressful life events. This is particularly striking during the year preceding surgery. The stresses noted include such items as major illness of a family member (44 percent), having to take a loan (26 percent), and death of a family member (18 percent) or of a close friend (18 percent). Sixteen percent have had a major weight gain (over 50 pounds) (Rand, Robbins, & Kaldau, 1983).

Patients' response to intestinal bypass surgery generally is positive (Andersen, Backer, Gudmand-Hoyer et al., 1979; Castelnuovo-Tedesco, 1980, 1982; Castelnuovo-Tedesco & Schiebel, 1976; Castelnuovo-Tedesco et al., 1982; Däno & Hahn-Pedersen, 1977; DeWind and Payne, 1976; Faloon, Flood, Aroesty et al., 1980; Halmi et al., 1980; Harris & Frame, 1968; Ishida, 1974; Kalucy et al., 1975; Mills & Stunkard, 1976; Solow, 1977; Solow, Silberfarb, & Swift, 1974). Somewhere between 66 and 90 percent of patients are pleased or very pleased with the results (Bray & Benfield, 1977; Scott et al., 1977). Although some investigators are more tentative than others (Abram et al., 1976; Crisp et al., 1977; Espmark, 1974; Kalucy & Crisp, 1974; Wise, 1976) and inclined to emphasize the occurrence of postoperative psychiatric difficulties, overall there is broad agreement that patients generally benefit psychologically from the operation. Däno and Hahn-Pedersen (1977) concluded that

> Jejunoileal bypass . . . in carefully informed and selected patients, stable in social and psychologic adjustment, can be performed without major psychiatric complications and results in improved working capacity, leisure time activity, sexual activity, and adjustment to daily life.

Studies of patients' emotional response to gastric bypass are not yet as numerous as those of the response to intestinal bypass, but the evidence so far indicates that the typical reaction is positive and that the results are consistent with those of jejuno-ileal bypass (Gomez, 1980; Halmi et al., 1980; Harris & Green, 1982; Mason et al., 1978; Saltzstein & Gutmann, 1980; Scott, 1982). Indeed, they are probably more favorable. Because serious metabolic complications generally do not occur after gastric bypass, the psychiatric consequences of protracted ill health are seen only exceptionally. On the other hand, a few patients are unable to adapt to the deprivation imposed by restricted food intake and may show substitutive symptoms, such as dependence on alcohol or drugs. Usually, however, there is a history of preoperative use of these substances.

The following description of the typical postoperative adaptive response is drawn largely from the literature on jejuno-ileal bypass, but it appears applicable to gastric bypass as well (with the exception, as mentioned, of the absence of psychiatric difficulties due to metabolic complications).

Almost immediately after surgery, patients begin to realize that they are steadily losing weight. Having battled obesity unsuccessfully for years, patients characteristically respond with great satisfaction and a sense of excitement as they see their fat steadily disappear. They consider this a real achievement and feel great relief (Castelnuovo-Tedesco, 1980; Castelnuovo-Tedesco & Schiebel, 1976; Däno & Hahn-Pedersen, 1977; Solow, 1977; Solow et al., 1974). They see their lives finally taking a positive turn and experience a feeling of being freed, at last, from the restrictions and limitations that for years obesity had imposed on them (Castelnuovo-Tedesco & Schiebel, 1976; Solow et al., 1974). In particular, they rediscover the pleasures of increased activity. This includes, first and foremost, physical activity, the capacity to walk without becoming fatigued or short of breath. Many had forgotten the joy of unhampered bodily movement. Somewhat later, patients also discover that they are becoming more active socially and that their responses to people are changing: They feel less shy and self-conscious and they mingle with others more freely. They are likely to report that they are taking steps toward finding employment (Castelnuovo-Tedesco, 1980; Castelnuovo-Tedesco & Schiebel, 1976; Däno & Hahn-Pedersen, 1977) and also that they are dating, perhaps for the first time in years, and becoming more active sexually. There is evidence, in other words, of increased self-confidence, of a lighter and more optimistic mood, of greater assertiveness, and of reappraisal of one's body size.

The main problems at this time have to do with a range of physical symptoms: diarrhea, nausea, and abdominal distress after eating. Weakness and vomiting may occur. Sometimes these have been looked on as "psychogenic" in origin; on the contrary, they usually are a manifestation of electrolyte or liver disturbances (the appearance of these symptoms should lead to prompt physical and laboratory examination of the patient) (Castelnuovo-Tedesco, 1980; Castelnuovo-Tedesco & Schiebel, 1976). It is well to remember that during this early period patients are so pleased with their weight loss that they may understate the occurrence of complications or may fail to report them altogether. The physician, therefore, needs to question these patients carefully to determine whether they may be experiencing more physical difficulties than they report spontaneously.

The next major milestone, usually after about six months, pertains to body size and physical activity. Patients rediscover that they can cross their legs, bend down and tie their shoelaces, sit in an ordinary armchair (which enables them to attend the movies or the theater), or pass through turnstiles at the supermarket. These are new accomplishments which the patient experiences with great pride and satisfaction. Another source of excitement is a new capacity to move about in public without eliciting attention or drawing comments from passersby. Some patients find this so invigorating that they say they have a sense of "being reborn."

Patients' experience with clothing further contributes to a new sense of pride and self-enhancement (Castelnuovo-Tedesco & Schiebel, 1976). They discover that they require progressively smaller sizes until finally they are able to resume shopping for ready-made clothes; this is extremely gratifying and like "a dream come true." At this point, women are inclined to select dresses that are more shapely and colorful than the ones they had worn prior to surgery. They also give more attention to grooming, use lipstick and other beauty aids, and generally look more attractive. They receive compliments about their appearance from family and friends and frequently they also have the experience, which is simultaneously exciting and disquieting, of not being recognized by an acquaintance during a casual encounter. These changes help to establish the patient's awareness of a "new self." Some patients discover that they can be the object of envy, often a new and pleasant surprise. For example, one patient noticed that her mother seemed envious of her new slimness; this culminated in the mother's decision to seek bypass surgery herself. Another aspect of patients' "new self" is their reluctance to mingle with obese people. This attitude surfaces approximately 6 months after surgery and becomes confirmed thereafter. Patients feel that associating with obese people interferes with the development of a "normal" identity. Also, they say, they do not like to be reminded of when *they* were obese.

Patients are also likely to report that they have become more outspoken, less concerned about pleasing others, and typically more assertive (Abram et al., 1976; Castelnuovo-Tedesco & Schiebel, 1976; Solow, 1977; Solow et al., 1974). They are pleased with these changes which contribute to improved self-esteem and to their positive view of the surgery.

Although the discussion so far has dwelt mainly on positive events and on adaptive gains and accomplishments, we need to keep in mind that this period is not devoid of stress (Abram et al., 1976; Castelnuovo-Tedesco & Schiebel, 1976; Kalucy & Crisp, 1974; Wise, 1976). This should not come as a surprise, inasmuch as patients lose almost half of their preoperative weight in the relatively brief time of approximately 1 year. Most patients become aware not only of enhanced self-esteem but also of greater emotionality and of fluctuations of anxiety, depression, and hostility (see Figures 11.3 and 11.4 based on responses to the multiple affect adjective checklist (Castelnuovo-Tedesco & Schiebel, 1976). They say they feel more in touch with all their feelings, positive and negative. Indeed, they appear more lively and responsive even though subjectively they may be more conscious of inner distress. Not infrequently patients spontaneously report that they have "developed quite a temper." This may raise tensions in their closest relationships, particularly those with spouses and parents. Marriages may become more strained and openly conflictual and may end in divorce (Abram et al., 1976; Castelnuovo-Tedesco, 1980; Kalucy & Crisp, 1974; Marshall & Neill, 1977; Neill, Marshall, & Yale, 1978). The divorce rate 3 years after intestinal bypass was somewhat higher than in a comparison group, particularly in those marriages originally found to be troubled before surgery

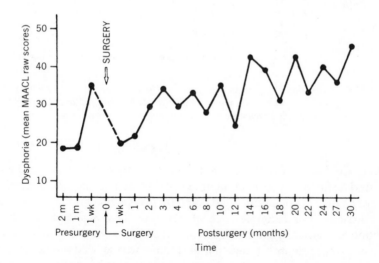

Figure 11.3. Composite picture of relative degree of dysphoria expressed by 10 bypass patients over 2.5 years. *Source:* Castelnuovo-Tedesco & Schiebel. (1976). Copyright 1976, the American Psychiatric Association. Reprinted by permission.

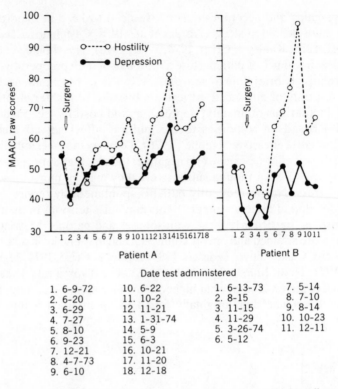

a: A score of 50 is the mean for a population of normal job applicants.

Figure 11.4. Fluctuations in level of self-reported depression and hostility for two bypass patients. *Source:* Castelnuovo-Tedesco & Schiebel. (1976). Copyright 1976, the American Psychiatric Association. Reprinted by permission.

(Rand, Kuldau, & Robbins, 1982). Yet, 69 percent of the surgical group reported a stable or improved marriage and greater sexual satisfaction. The issue of change in appearance and body size plays a direct role in the status of the marriage. For example, one of our patients was abandoned by her husband immediately prior to her scheduled bypass operation; her husband (who was thin) promptly found himself another woman who was fat. Another of our patients postoperatively became intolerant of the appearance of her husband, who was also superobese. Her attitude finally prompted him to seek bypass surgery, but the operation did not repair the strain in the marriage, which culminated in divorce. Patients who are single or recently divorced may experience stress when they begin dating actively. This is felt especially when expectations of closeness or permanence are added to these new relationships (Castelnuovo-Tedesco, 1980, 1982; Castelnuovo-Tedesco & Schiebel, 1976). One of our patients postoperatively had her first sexual encounter which she found enjoyable and gratifying; however, she became acutely anxious when her boyfriend "became serious" and proposed marriage. Other women patients also seemed comfortable as long as they could regard a new relationship as a temporary "affair," but became distressed when their partners began to reveal expectations of permanence and commitment. They particularly wished to avoid anything that they perceived as binding. This attitude was forcibly expressed by one patient who said, "Love is something between two people, like handcuffs" (Castelnuovo-Tedesco & Schiebel, 1975, 1976).

An issue not fully resolved is that of postoperative psychiatric complications. Some investigators have conveyed the view that serious reactions, primarily depressions, occur not infrequently (Abram et al., 1976; Espmark, 1974; Kalucy and Crisp, 1974; Wise, 1976). Generally, however, these authors have not adequately described these depressions or the circumstances surrounding them, leaving the impression that these were "psychogenic" disturbances in response to the stress of the operation or of weight loss. Espmark (1974), for example, reports that of his 65 patients 40 needed postoperative psychotherapy "due to anxiety and depression," 3 had "serious psychogenic vomiting," 4 made "serious suicidal attempts," and that 17 had "reported thoughts of suicide or weariness of life." Other patients experienced what Espmark calls "crises of self assertion" and "body image crises." Espmark, unfortunately, gives no details about his patients' physical condition at the time when they were experiencing these psychiatric complications; one wonders if these difficulties were not an expression of their encounter with severe ill health. Other psychiatric authors (Abram et al., 1976; Crisp et al., 1977; Wise, 1976) also have tended to give little notice to patients' complex metabolic difficulties; diarrhea is the physical problem mainly emphasized, while the other postoperative complications, which are much more serious and by no means uncommon, are hardly mentioned. As reported elsewhere (Castelnuovo-Tedesco, 1980, 1982; Castelnuovo-Tedesco & Schiebel, 1976) even though rapid weight loss may be experienced as somewhat stressful and accompanied by mood fluctuations, severe depressions rarely occur on this basis alone. To be specific, I have not seen major postoperative psychiatric decompensations in bypass patients except in the context and as a consequence of protracted physical difficulties.

When carefully interviewed, these patients make it very clear that their emotional distress, in some cases marked, is occurring because they are very ill. Patients especially refer to their ill health, which they find frightening and destabilizing. It is not difficult to appreciate that after weeks, months, and occasionally years of debilitating or painful physical symptoms these patients can, and do, become very depressed and discouraged, at times suicidal. It is important to bear in mind that these patients, prior to their operation, typically had enjoyed robust good health and never had been hospitalized. As a consequence, the experience of protracted ill health following surgery is especially frightening. These feelings are compounded by the realization that the treatment of some of the major complications of intestinal bypass surgery (e.g., bypass enteritis, hepatitis) is not yet fully established and that physicians at times have difficulty controlling them (Castelnuovo-Tedesco, 1980). Also, patients who do not live near the medical center where the operation was performed sometimes discover that their hometown physician may be unfamiliar with the complications of bypass surgery and unsure about how to treat them. For example, one patient, who had had recurrent episodes of shaking chills and high fever (due to bypass enteritis), repeatedly had consulted her physician but had been told not to worry and that "it was nothing, just the flu." Finally, upset about not receiving effective help, she had returned to the medical center where her symptoms were identified as complications of the jejuno-ileal bypass and treated appropriately.

Patients with repeated vomiting may find that the physiologic basis (electrolyte disturbance or bypass enteritis) remains undiagnosed; the symptom may be considered "psychogenic" (Starkloff, Donovan, Ramach et al., 1975). Thus, a patient of ours whose depression and anxiety were associated with progressive renal insufficiency and increasing ill health, had been referred in his hometown for intensive psychotherapy, while his worsening physical condition had gone unrecognized and untreated.

Reoperation may become necessary, if serious physical symptoms persist. Several options are available. Reversal of the bypass (with reestablishment of normal intestinal continuity) or revision of the bypass (with exteriorization of the end of the jejunal loop) may be carried out. More recently, reversal of the bypass has been combined with a gastric bypass. Reversal of the jejuno-ileal bypass may be life saving and becomes necessary in 8 to 25 percent of cases (Halverson, Scheff, Gentry et al., 1980; Scott, 1982). A striking finding is that, when the bypass has been reversed, the emotional as well as the physical symptoms usually subside promptly (Reynolds, 1978; Wise, 1976). Patients, however, then encounter a new set of problems: They regain their original weight and this, typically, brings renewed misery and discouragement. For this reason, in the last few years the usual approach has been to convert an inadequate intestinal bypass (due to insufficient absorption reduction) or a malfunctioning intestinal bypass (with associated toxic complications) into a gastric bypass (Mason et al., 1980; Halverson et al., 1981). In both instances, this usually has proven very satisfactory.

Patients' Attitudes toward Bypass Procedures

Most patients maintain a positive attitude toward the bypass procedures, even in cases where serious complications have occurred (Bray & Benfield, 1977; Castelnuovo-Tedesco, 1980, 1982; Castelnuovo-Tedesco & Schiebel, 1976; Castelnuovo-Tedesco et al., 1982; Faloon et al., 1980). This holds true even when reoperation has been necessary. A recent study of the long-term adjustment to jejuno-ileal bypass, showed that most patients (79 percent) were positive about the operation and pleased to recommend it to others, although some (29 percent) expressed reservations and were cautious in recommending it. Thirteen percent were distinctly ambivalent and 8 percent were highly dissatisfied and outspokenly opposed to the operation. Also of interest is, that following jejuno-ileal bypass, most patients (92 percent) had maintained or increased their school or work effectiveness and achievement; only 8 percent had worsened (Castelnuovo-Tedesco et al., 1982). Such accomplishments of course contribute to patients' positive view of the operation (as one patient put it, "You can stand almost anything as long as you are losing weight"). According to another study (Kuldau & Rand, 1980), "91 percent of the patients said they would probably or definitely have the operation again, knowing what they now knew."

A notable finding is that patients often use denial in assessing their surgical experience; at times it is extreme (Castelnuovo-Tedesco, 1980, 1982; Castelnuovo-Tedesco et al., 1982). For example, a physician who, after intestinal bypass surgery, was having serious electrolyte problems, referred one of his own patients for bypass surgery; the latter, parenthetically, did much better than the physician. If the quest for intestinal bypass has been a disappointment, patients have trouble acknowledging it. They are reluctant to conclude that the original decision may have been a mistake or that they may require further surgery. A striking finding is the willingness of these patients to endure ill health from bypass complications for months or even years before they will agree to a reversal of the bypass (Castelnuovo-Tedesco, 1980, 1982). They are pleased with their weight loss, even though it may have been purchased at the cost of new, and sometimes serious, health problems. They are fearful—with justification—that if they undergo reversal of the bypass they will once more gain weight to their preoperative level. (This, as has been noted, can now be avoided by converting the intestinal bypass into a gastric bypass.)

The prominence of denial is a critical issue which influences, from the very beginning, the physician's contact with these patients and their response to the operation (Castelnuovo-Tedesco, 1980; Castelnuovo-Tedesco et al., 1982). First, preoperatively, even when one tries conscientiously to inform the patient about the operation, its consequences and possible complications, one may note that the patient has not heard fully what he or she needs to hear. In short, in these cases "informed consent" is no simple matter. For this reason, we have suggested that at least a month elapse between the patient's first contact with the surgical team and the operation, and that during this time the patient be spoken to repeatedly, preferably by more than one person (Castelnuovo-Tedesco, 1982; Castelnuovo-Tedesco & Schiebel, 1976). This waiting period also facilitates the task of identifying those persons who are doubtful candidates for the procedure on psychiatric grounds (the poorly motivated, the insufficiently cooperative, the impulsive, and the emotionally fragile). In a similar vein, according to Stellar and Rodin (1980), "one surgeon tests his patients on what they've agreed on and postpones treatment if they fail the test."

Another aspect of the denial problem is that patients who fail to return for regular follow-up have more complications, medical and psychiatric (Castelnuovo-Tedesco et al., 1982; Leon et al., 1979).

Finally, denial influences efforts to obtain objective assessments of bypass surgery, since these are based in large measure on patients' report of their satisfaction with the results. Patients' tendency to understate negative experiences produces assessments that are skewed artificially toward the positive (Castelnuovo-Tedesco et al., 1982).

CONCLUSIONS

Intestinal and gastric bypass operations are interesting medical developments in several respects. They attempt to deal radically with a condition of highly complex etiology because the specific etiologic factors are not under our direct therapeutic control. They also represent the willingness to use far-reaching surgical means electively to improve the quality of the patient's life. Although fear of a shortened life span and of future medical problems play a large role in the quest for bypass surgery, the patient's principal motive is to reduce the burden caused by obesity and to normalize his or her life (Solow et al., 1974). This includes more than purely cosmetic considerations. The latter, in fact, play a decidedly minor *conscious* role (Castelnuovo-Tedesco & Schiebel, 1976; Hutzler et al., 1981). To grasp the motives for seeking bypass surgery, we should bear in mind that most who undergo these procedures are young, in good health, and generally have no immediate physical difficulties, apart from the obesity itself. Also, unlike other medical conditions, obesity is not painful and does not directly interfere with vital functions. Nonetheless, patients feel so strongly about their handicap that they are willing to undergo a major surgical procedure. The latter, though usually successful or at least relatively successful, occasionally has remarkably poor results. In short, we are struck by the intensity of these patients' wish to normalize their lives and, by inference, by the emotional burden that obesity entails (Solow et al., 1974). We are struck also by how far patients use denial to sustain and justify their decision on behalf of surgery, even when the result has been mediocre or worse (Castelnuovo-Tedesco, 1980; Castelnuovo-Tedesco et al., 1982).

For these reasons, controversy concerning these procedures continues, even though they have been used for about 25 years and results have steadily improved, especially since the introduction of gastric bypass. On the one hand, they are performed in great numbers and may be described in every sense as popular operations, on the other their status is not yet resolved because of the occasional occurrence of very serious complications which, as yet, are difficult to predict or prevent. Thus, there are some who continue to regard them as experimental procedures (Andersen et al., 1979; Hirsch, 1974; Ravitch & Brolin, 1979), and some who oppose them on fundamental grounds (Wooley, Wooley, & Dyrenforth, 1980). Some still retain a fragment of the thought that the patient ought to be able to exercise the self-discipline necessary to lose weight on his or her own. For example, a recent editorial in a major medical journal offered the judgement that superobese patients who opt for surgery "seek a cure for an ailment for which they are unwilling to accept any responsibility" (Alpers, 1983). We are faced, at any rate, with a paradox: these operations have achieved a high degree of acceptance among patients, but have not yet received the unqualified approval of investigators in this field.

A final comment: Despite their limitations, these procedures still are the most effective available treatment for a disorder that is essentially unresponsive to conservative methods and that, otherwise, results in progressively grave handicap and risk.

REFERENCES

Abram, H. S., Meixel, S. A., Webb, W. W., et al. (1976). Psychological adaptation to jejunoileal bypass for morbid obesity. *Journal of Nervous and Mental Diseases, 162;* 151–157.

Alpers, D. H. (1983). Surgical therapy for obesity. *New England Journal of Medicine, 308* (17); 1026–1027.

Andersen, B., Backer, O., Gudmand-Hoyer, E. et al. (1979). Randomized trial of jejunoileal bypass versus medical treatment in morbid obesity. The Danish obesity project. *Lancet, 2* (8155); 1255–1258.

Atkinson, R. M., & Ringuette, E. L. (1967). A survey of biographical and psychological features in extraordinary fatness. *Psychosomatic Medicine, 29* (2); 121–133.

Bray, G. A., & Benfield, J. R. (1977). Intestinal bypass for obesity: A summary and perspective. *American Journal of Clinical Nutrition, 30;* 121–127.

Bray, G. A., Dahms, W. T., & Atkinson, R. L. et al. (1980). Factors controlling food intake: A comparison of dieting and intestinal bypass. *American Journal of Nutrition, 33;* 376–382.

Bray, G. A., Zachary, B., Dahms, W. T. et al. (1978). Eating patterns of the massively obese individuals. *Journal of American Dietic Association, 72;* 24–27.

Bruch, H. (1952). Psychological aspects of reducing. *Psychosomatic Medicine, 14;* 337–346.

Bruch, H. (1957). *The Importance of Overweight.* New York: Norton.

Bruch, H. (1973). *Eating Disorders.* New York: Basic.

Buchwald, H. (1980). True informed consent in surgical treatment of morbid obesity: The current case for both jejunoileal and gastric bypass. *American Journal of Clinical Nutrition, 33;* 482–494.

Buckwalter, J. A., & Herbst, C. A. (1980). Complications of gastric bypass for morbid obesity. *American Journal of Surgery, 139;* 55–60.

Bychowski, G. (1950). On neurotic obesity. *Psychoanalytic Review, 37* (4); 301–319.

Castelnuovo-Tedesco, P. (1980). Jejunoileal bypass for superobesity: A psychiatric assessment. *Advances in Psychosomatic Medicine, 10;* 196–206.

Castelnuovo-Tedesco, P. (1982). Surgical treatment of obesity: Psychiatric aspects. In M. Zales (Ed.), *Eating, Sleeping and Sexuality.* New York: Brunner Mazel.

Castelnuovo-Tedesco, P., Buchanan, D. C., & Hall, H. D. (1980). Jaw wiring for obesity. *General Hospital Psychiatry, 2;* 156–159.

Castelnuovo-Tedesco, P., & Schiebel, D. (1975). Studies of superobesity. I. Psychological characteristics of superobese patients. *International Journal of Psychiatry in Medicine, 6;* 465–480.

Castelnuovo-Tedesco, P., & Schiebel, D. (1976). Studies of superobesity. II. Psychiatric appraisal of jejunoileal bypass surgery. *American Journal of Psychiatry, 133;* 26–31.

Castelnuovo-Tedesco, P., Weinberg, J., & Buchanan, D. C. et al. (1982). Long-term outcome of jejunoileal bypass surgery for superobesity: A psychiatric assessment. *American Journal of Psychiatry, 139* (10); 1248–1252.

Charles, S. C., Blumberg, P., Mozello, J. et al. (in press). Psychiatric diagnosis in candidates for gastroplasty. *International Journal of Eating Disorders.*

Crisp, A. H., Kalucy, R. S., Pilkington, T. R. E. et al. (1977). Some psychological consequences of ileojejunal bypass surgery. *American Journal of Clinical Nutrition, 30;* 109–120.

Däno, P., & Hahn-Pedersen, J. (1977). Improvement in quality of life following jejunoileal bypass surgery for obesity. *Scandinavian Journal of Gastroenterology, 12;* 769–774.

DeWind, L. T., & Payne, J. H. (1976). Intestinal bypass surgery for morbid obesity: Longterm results. *Journal of the American Medical Association, 236;* 2298–2301.

Engel, G. L. (1955). Studies of ulcerative colitis. III. The nature of the psychologic processes. *American Journal of Medicine, 19* (2); 231–256.

Espmark, S. (1974). *Psychological adjustment before and after bypass surgery for extreme obesity—A preliminary report.* First International Congress on Obesity, London.

Faloon, W. W. (1977). Ileal bypass for obesity: Postoperative perspective. *Hospital Practice, 12;* 73–82.

Faloon, W. W. Flood, M. S., Aroesty, S. et al. (1980). Assessment of jejunoileostomy for obesity — some observations since 1976. *American Journal of Clinical Nutrition, 33;* 431–439.

Fink, G., Gottesfeld, H., & Glickman, L. (1962). The "superobese" patient. *Journal of Hillside Hospital, 11;* 97–119.

Garrow, J. S. (1980). Combined medical-surgical approaches to treatment of obesity. *American Journal of Clinical Nutrition, 33;* 425–430.

Gaspar, M. R., Movius, H. J., Rosental, J. J. et al (1976). Comparison of Payne and Scott operations for morbid obesity. *Annals of Surgery, 184;* 507–515.

Gomez, C. A. (1980). Gastroplasty in the surgical treatment of morbid obesity. *American Journal of Clinical Nutrition, 33;* 406–415.

Hallberg, D. (1980). A survey of surgical techniques for treatment of obesity and a remark on the bilio-intestinal bypass method. *American Journal of Clinical Nutrition, 33;* 499–501.

Halmi, K. A., Long, M., Stunkard, A. J. et al. (1980). Psychiatric diagnosis of morbidly obese gastric bypass patients. *American Journal of Psychiatry, 137* (4); 470–472.

Halmi, K. A., Mason, E., Falk, J. et al. (1981). Appetitive behavior after gastric bypass for obesity. *International Journal of Obesity, 5* (5); 457–464.

Halmi, K. A., Stunkard, A. J., & Mason, E. E. (1980). Emotional responses to weight reduction by three methods: Gastric bypass, jejunoileal bypass, diet. *American Journal of Clinical Nutrition, 33;* 446–451.

Halverson, J. D., Scheff, R. J., Gentry, K. et al. (1980). Long-term follow-up of jejunoileal bypass patients. *American Journal of Clinical Nutrition, 33;* 472–475.

Halverson, J. D., Zuckerman, G. R., Koehler, R. E. et al. (1981). Gastric bypass for morbid obesity. A medical-surgical assessment. *Annals of Surgery, 194* (2); 152–160.

Hamburger, W. W. (1951). Emotional aspects of obesity. *Medical Clinics of North America, 35;* 483–499.

Harris, J., & Frame, B. (1968). *A psychiatric study of patients undergoing intestinal bypass for treatment of intractable obesity.* 121st Annual Meeting of American Psychiatric Association. Boston, MA.

Harris, M. B., & Green, D. (1982). Psychosocial effects of gastric reduction surgery for obesity. *International Journal of Obesity, 7;* 527–539.

Hecht, M. B. (1955). Obesity in women; A psychiatric study. *Psychiatric Quarterly, 29;* 203–231.

Hirsch, J. (1974). Jejunoileal shunt for obesity. *New England Journal of Medicine, 190;* 962–963.

Holland, J., Masling, J., & Copley, D. (1970). Mental illness in lower class normal, obese and hyperobese women. *Psychosomatic Medicine, 32;* 351–357.

Hutzler, J. C., Keen, J., Molinari, V. et al. (1981). Superobesity: A psychiatric profile of patients electing gastric stapling for the treatment of morbid obesity. *Journal of Clinical Psychiatry, 42* (12); 458–462.

Ishida, Y. (1974). Sexuality after small bowel bypass. *Current Medical Dialogues, 41;* 659–662.

Kalucy, R. S., & Crisp, A. H. (1974). Some psychological and social implications of massive obesity. *Journal of Psychosomatic Research, 18;* 465–473.

Kalucy, R. S., Solow, C., Hartmann, M. et al. (1975). Self reports of estimated body widths in female obese subjects with major fat loss following ileojejunal bypass surgery. In A. Howard, (Ed.), *Recent Advances in Obesity Research. Proceedings of the First International Congress on Obesity* (pp. 331–333). London: Newman.

Kark, A. E. (1980). Jaw wiring. *American Journal of Clinical Nutrition, 33;* 420–424.

Kollar, E. J., & Atkinson, R. M. (1966). Responses of extremely obese patients to starvation. *Psychosomatic Medicine, 28;* 227–246.

Kollar E. J., Atkinson, R. M., & Albin, D. L. (1969). The effectiveness of fasting in the treatment of superobesity. *Psychosomatics, 10;* 125–135.

Kuldau, M. J., & Rand, C. S. W. (1980). Jejunoileal bypass: General and psychiatric outcome after one year. *Psychosomatics, 21* (7); 534–539.

Leon, G. R., Eckert, E. D., Teed, D. et al. (1979). Changes in body image and other psychological factors after intestinal bypass surgery for massive obesity. *Journal of Behavioral Medicine, 2* (1); 39–55.

Marshall, J. R., & Neill, J. (1977). The removal of a psychosomatic symptom: Effects on the marriage. *Family Process, 16* (3); 273–280.

Mason, E. E., & Ito, C. (1969). Gastric bypass. *Annals of Surgery, 170;* 329–339.

Mason, E. E., Printen, K. J., Blommers, T. J. et al. (1978). Gastric bypass for obesity after ten years experience. *International Journal of Obesity, 2;* 197–206.

Mason, E. E., Printen, K. J., Blommers, T. J. et al. (1980). Gastric bypass in morbid obesity. *American Journal of Clinical Nutrition, 33;* 395–405.

Mendelson, M., Weinberg, N., & Stunkard, A. J. (1961). Obesity in men: A clinical study of twenty five cases. *Annals of International Medicine, 54;* 660–671.

Meyer, J. E., & Tuchelt-Gallwiz, A. (1963). A study on social image, body image and the problem of psychogenetic factors in obesity. *Comprehensive Psychiatry, 9* (2); 148–154.

Mills, M. J., & Stunkard, A. J. (1976). Behavioral changes following surgery for obesity. *American Journal of Psychiatry, 133;* 527–531.

Neill, J. R., & Marshall, J. R. (1976). End-to-end jejunoileal bypass for morbid obesity: The psychosocial outcome. *Wisconsin Medical Journal, 76;* 103–105.

Neill, J. R., Marshall, J. R., & Yale, C. E. (1978). Marital changes after intestinal bypass surgery. *Journal of the American Medical Association, 240;* 447–450.

Payne, J. H., DeWind, L. T., Commons, R. R. (1963). Metabolic observations in patients with jejunocolic shunts. *American Journal of Surgery, 106;* 273–289.

Phillips, R. B. (1978). Small intestinal bypass for the treatment of morbid obesity. *Surgery of Gynecology and Obstetrics, 146;* 455–468.

Pi-Sunyer, F. X. (1976). Jejunoileal bypass surgery for obesity. *American Journal of Clinical Nutrition, 29;* 409–416.

Rand, C. W., Kuldau, M. J., & Robbins, L. (1982). Surgery for obesity and marriage quality. *Journal of the American Medical Association, 247* (10); 1419–1422.

Rand, C. W., Robbins, L., & Kuldau, J. M. (1983). Stressful life events and the decision for surgery for obesity. *Psychosomatics, 24* (4); 377–384.

Rascovsky, A., deRascovsky, M. W., Schlossberg, T. (1950). Basic psychic structure of the obese. *International Journal of Psycho-Analysis, 31;* 144–149.

Ravitch, M. M., & Brolin, R. E. (1979). The price of weight loss by jejunoileal shunt. *Annals of Surgery, 190;* 382–391.

Reivich, R. S., Ruiz, R. A., & Lapi, R. M. (1966). Extreme obesity. *Journal of the Kansas Medical Society, 67;* 134–140.

Reynolds, T. B. (1978). Medical complications of intestinal bypass surgery. In G. H. Stollerman, (Ed.), *Advances in Internal Medicine (Vol. 23, pp. 47–59).* Chicago: Year Book Medical Publications.

Richardson, H. B. (1946). Obesity and neurosis. *Psychiatric Quarterly, 20;* 400–424.

Rodin, J. (1976). The relationship between external responsiveness and the development and maintenance of obesity. In Novin, D., Wyrwicka, W. & Gray, G.

(Eds.). *Hunger: Basic Mechanisms and Clinical Implications* (pp. 409–419). New York: Raven.

Rodin, J. (1980). Changes in perceptual responsiveness following jejuno-ileostomy: Their potential role in reducing food intake. *American Journal of Clinical Nutrition, 33;* 457–464.

Saltzstein, E. C., & Gutmann, M. C. (1980). Gastric bypass for morbid obesity. Preoperative and postoperative psychological evaluation of patients. *Archives of Surgery, 115;* 21–28.

Schiebel, D., & Castelnuovo-Tedesco, P. (1978). Studies of superobesity: III. Body image changes after jejunoileal bypass surgery. *International Journal of Psychiatry in Medicine, 8;* 117–123.

Sclafani, A. (1981). Appetitive behavior after jejunoileal bypass. *International Journal of Obesity, 5;* 449–455.

Scott, H. W. Jr. (1982). Jejunoileal bypass versus gastric bypass or gastroplasty in the operative treatment of obesity. *Langenbeck's Archiv für Chirurgie, 356;* 25–35.

Scott, H. W. Jr., Dean, Rother, Shull, J. H. et al. (1977). Results of jejuno-ileal bypass in two hundred patients with morbid obesity. *Surgery of Gynecology and Obstetrics, 145;* 661–673.

Solow, C. (1977). Psychosocial aspects of intestinal bypass for massive obesity: Current status. *American Journal of Clinical Nutrition, 30;* 103–108.

Solow, C., Silberfarb, P. M., & Swift, K. (1974). Psychosocial effects of intestinal bypass surgery for severe obesity. *New England Journal of Medicine, 290;* 300–304.

Starkloff, G. B., Donovan, J. F., Ramach, R. et al. (1975). Metabolic intestinal surgery. Its complications and management. *Archives of Metabolic Surgery, 11;* 652–657.

Stellar, J. E., & Rodin, J. (1980). Workshop III. Research needs. *American Journal of Clinical Nutrition, 33;* 526–527.

Stunkard, A., & Burt, V. (1967). Obesity and the body image: II. Age at onset of disturbances of the body image. *American Journal of Psychiatry, 123;* 1443–1447.

Stunkard, A. J. (1957). The "dieting depression." *American Journal of Medicine, 23;* 77–86.

Stunkard, A. J. (1959). Eating patterns and obesity. *Psychiatric Quarterly, 33;* 284–295.

Stunkard, A. J., Grace, W. J., & Wolff, H. G. (1955). The night-eating syndrome: A pattern of food intake among certain obese patients. *American Journal of Medicine, 19;* 78–86.

Stunkard, A., & McLaren-Hume, H. (1959). The results of treatment for obesity. *Archives of International Medicine, 103;* 79–85.

Stunkard, A., & Mendelson, M. (1961). Disturbances in body image of some obese persons. *Journal of the American Dietetic Association, 38;* 328–331.

Stunkard, A., & Mendelson, M. (1967). Obesity and the body image: I. Characteristics of disturbances in the body image of some obese persons. *American Journal of Psychiatry, 123;* 1296–1300.

Swanson, D. W., & Dinello, F. A. (1970). Severe obesity as a habituation syndrome: Evidence during a starvation study. *Archives of General Psychiatry. 22;* 120–127.

Van Itallie, T. B. (1980). Morbid obesity: A hazardous disorder that resists conservative treatment. *American Journal of Clinical Nutrition 33;* 358–363.

Webb, W. W., Phares, R., Abram H. S. et al. (1976). Jejunoileal bypass procedures in morbid obesity; preoperative psychological findings. *Journal of Clinical Psychology, 32;* 82–85.

Weinberg, N., Mendelson, M., & Stunkard, A. (1961). A failure to find distinctive personality features in a group of obese men. *American Journal of Psychiatry, 117;* 1035–1037.

Werkman, S. L., & Greenberg, E. S. (1967). Personality and interest patterns in obese adolescent girls. *Psychosomatic Medicine, 29;* 72–80.

Wise, T. N. (1976). Adverse psychologic reactions to ileal bypass surgery. *Southern Medical Journal, 69;* 1533–1535.

Wise, T. N., & Fernandez, F. (1979). Psychological profiles of candidates seeking surgical correction for obesity. *Obesity/Bariatric Medicine, 8* (3); 83–86.

Wooley, S. C., Wooley, O. W., & Dyrenforth, S. (1980). The case against radical interventions. *American Journal of Clinical Nutrition, 33;* 465–471.

Wulff, M. (1932). Über einen interessanten oralen Symptomen-Komplex und seine Beziehung zur Sucht. *Internationale Zeitschrift für Psychoanalyse, 18* (3); 181–203.

— CHAPTER TWELVE

Cosmetic Surgery, with Particular Reference to Rhinoplasty

LOUIS LINN, M.D.

Cosmetic surgery may be described as an optional procedure designed to make essentially normal people look better. It has been estimated that close to one-half million such procedures were carried out in 1984 by over 2700 surgeons who are certified in this field. These operations included procedures on the breast for augmentation, reduction and lifting; blepharoplasty; rhinoplasty; rhitidectomy (face lift); suction lipectomy; dermabrasion and chemical skin peeling; abdominoplasty; mentoplasty; otoplasty; hair transplants; and body contour alterations. The incidence of cosmetic procedures has gone up by over 60 percent between 1981 and 1984. New procedures have evolved, such as the use of lasers to remove birth marks and suction lipectomy to remove regional fat accumulations. In general, surgical techniques have improved greatly and good results are more reliably obtainable. Other changes in the field include a sharp rise in the number of men applying for cosmetic surgery. In the past decade, men have gone from perhaps 5 percent of plastic surgery patients to somewhere around 20 percent (Clark et al., 1985).

In recent years there has been a growing emphasis on the common sense approach to cosmetic surgery, namely, that improved appearance can be profoundly psychotherapeutic. (Berscheid and Gangestad, 1982; DeMoura, 1978; Goin, Burgoyne, Goin, & Staples, 1980; Groenman and Sauer, 1983; Jensen, 1978; Macgregor, 1982a and 1982b, pp. 283 – 288, 387 – 398). A psychoanalytic preoccupation which demands that the patient learn to make peace with his appearance is often in error. The author can recall several patients from the past with whom he conducted long and frustrating psychoanalyses that would have been facilitated and shortened if a reasonable request for cosmetic surgery had been acceded to.

It is often difficult to evaluate the degree to which environmental factors or purely internal psychological factors predominate in a given case. Usually, we are dealing with a dialogue in which certain environments are more of a problem in this regard, and others are less demanding. In the long run, it is the patient's *unhappiness* with the fit between himself and the environment which is the basis for his request for cosmetic surgery. In this sense it is a fallacy to try to avoid the "emotionally disturbed" cosmetic surgery candidate (Linn & Goldman, 1949).

THE PROBLEM OF RHINOPLASTY

My own interest in this subject began on my return to civilian life after World War II. I was on the psychiatric staff of Mount Sinai Hospital in New York City and wanted to study the problem of experimental psychosis. This was in 1946, in what you might call the pre-psychedelic days, that is, before hallucinogenic substances became freely available as street drugs and gave us many more opportunities than we now want to observe psychotic reactions in *statu nascendi*. I recalled my medical school teachings which warned against the psychologic dangers of rhinoplasty. "Patients may become obsessed with a minor nasal deformity," we were told, "which was acting psychologically as a crutch. These patients tend to attribute all their social woes," this explanation continued, "to this clearly inconsequential imperfection and by removing it we deprive these unfortunate patients of an essential defense mechanism, and this could collapse the entire emotional adaptational system with a resulting psychotic reaction." A patient with a psychotic illness which started soon after rhinoplasty would then be presented to the medical students. The presentation was dramatic and the lesson seemed clear. "Beware of rhinoplasty unless your patient has had a careful psychiatric clearance!"

When I learned that we had a rhinoplasty clinic at Mount Sinai Hospital, I felt I was in luck. This seemed precisely the setting I was looking for, in which I could observe emerging acute psychotic reactions by the score. I worked with Dr. Irving Goldman, a distinguished surgeon who headed up the rhinoplasty clinic, and together we collected our data. In 1949 we published a paper (Linn & Goldman). It covered pre- and postoperative observations as well as a 6-month follow up on 74 rhinoplasty patients. All patients with a clearly correctable nasal deformity received surgery, regardless of the psychiatric diagnosis. It was my opinion then that every patient we saw had some degree of psychopathology, ranging at one extreme from mild neurotic reactions of anxiety and depression to chronic schizophrenic reactions which started years before the surgery at the other. In not a single case in our series was the psychiatric disorder made worse. In many cases the psychiatric improvement was unmistakable, and I will describe them later. For the moment let me say that my initial chagrin at not seeing many acute psychotic reactions soon gave way to the realization that the gloomy view I learned in school was wrong, that rhinoplasty was not dangerous, that it was an essentially benign procedure from a psychiatric point of view. Acute postoperative disturbances do occur from time to time and psychiatric judgment must be exercised in all cases. However, the incidence of these severe psychiatric complications was clearly low. In 1949 when our rhinoplasty paper was published it is estimated that there were approximately 15,000 rhinoplasty procedures in that year in the United States. By 1971 the number had climbed to several hundred thousands. In the decade and a half since then the number of procedures per year has increased still further. In this time surgical skills have improved immensely. The surgical message is unchanged from that we expressed in 1949, namely, that the incidence of serious psychiatric complications following rhinoplasty remains very low.

HOW RHINOPLASTY HELPS

Most of our cases were women. Among them we found a characteristic set of symptoms which we called the "rhinoplasty syndrome." It is not meant as a joke to say that these patients did all they could to preserve a low profile. In public settings they tried to avoid side views of the nose. They dressed plainly. They avoided the use of jewelry. Hair styles and hats were selected to achieve inconspicuousness and anonymity. Because they were chronically and painfully aware of the nose in profile, they adopted various mannerisms with the hands calculated to cover the nose. They were often awkward in their manner and distracted in their thoughts so that they functioned at a distinct disadvantage in social settings.

It is easy to understand why an unconventional or nonconforming nasal configuration can cause emotional discomfort. The nose is a maximally conspicuous structure from a social point of view. In the sensorimotor map of a human cerebral cortex, the representation of the nose along with the rest of the face occupies an extraordinarily high fraction of the total body area. Thus, its neuro-physiological connections are vast and its psychological significance correspondingly complex. In addition, the nose is the repository of clearcut sexual symbolism (Book, 1971). There is a striking difference in the appearance of a large strong male nose and the delicate contours of a female nose. Thus, the nasal configuration helps define the message of masculinity or femininity which the patient transmits to others. There are some women who are attractively feminine in all their physical characteristics except for the nose. These women often complain (correctly), "This is my father's nose. It looks good on him, not on me." Apart from the esthetic issues that are at stake, there are strong symbolic issues because such a nasal configuration may complicate an already shaky problem revolving about normal adult sexual identity. As indicated earlier, years of struggle in psycho-analytically oriented psychotherapy may be bypassed by the simple device of surgical correction. On a more superficial note, there are Hollywood-created stereotypes to which a woman may want to conform. In any case, an unattractive nose can reduce a woman's self-esteem.

Self-esteem is to the psychiatrist what hemoglobin is to the hematologist. The patient must have a certain adequate level of self-esteem for successful social functioning. Acquiring a nasal configuration that the patient likes and that generates pride is a powerful device for enhancing self-esteem. This in turn can create a "ripple effect" that reverses the rhinoplasty syndrome. Postoperatively the patient tends to dress more attractively. She arranges her hair more boldly. She uses jewelry and cosmetics more freely. In short, she becomes more relaxed in her social behavior. The effect of all this is to elicit a more positive response from the environment. This may result in profound changes in the quantity and quality of a patient's social interactions.

SHORT-TERM VERSUS LONG-TERM OUTCOME

The foregoing short-term changes tend to occur over a period of months as the postoperative edema and the ecchymoses subside. The majority of the patients experience a sense of elation and rebirth into a more friendly social world. As the wheels of social activity spin faster, however, new problems may emerge associated with dating, sexual involvements, courtship, marriage, parenting, and so forth. These new problems often require the help of a psychotherapist. Thus, while a successful surgical result can of itself be of immense psychotherapeutic value, direct psychiatric help may also be advisable. It should be noted at this point that the patient who has been socially activated by the procedure is easier to treat psychotherapeutically than the patient who is in a state of social withdrawal and who is mono-maniacally obsessed with the shape of the nose.

A curious phenomenon which is sometimes observed during the post-operative period is a tendency to nasal self-injury. "Accidentally" the patient may bump into the door of the medicine chest or into the windshield of the car in a minor automobile accident. The nose may be broken in these incidents and, in effect, a nasal deformity is reestablished.

There are some curious long-term effects of rhinoplasty. A wife may fail to disclose to her husband that she had cosmetic surgery before they met. The birth of a baby may activate a fear that the child may inherit the "bad" nose. This concern may contribute to a postpartum emotional upheaval. In addition, an immature narcissistic woman who was perhaps functioning adequately as long as she was the sole object of her husband's attentions may break down postpartum because of her inability to function as a mother. These long-term complications emphasize the fact that the surgically induced emotional improvements may have to be supplemented with psycho-analytically oriented psychotherapy in selected cases. Many patients who come for rhinoplasty are not introspectively inclined and may be unwilling to accept a recommendation for supplementary psychotherapeutic help. Even in these cases, however, the long-term psychiatric prognosis is generally good where a clearly correctable nasal deformity exists.

Having emphasized the overall good prognosis in most rhinoplasty cases, it is necessary to note the fact that with the best surgical care and psycho-logical scrutiny, a small group of cases will decompensate postoperatively. These patients and their families will plague the surgeon and sue the surgeon. The impact on him may be so traumatic that he will never forget it. Therefore more should be said about these cases.

THE BODY IMAGE CONCEPT

In trying to comprehend the problems of the rhinoplasty patient, it is useful to refer to Schilder's "Body Image" concept (Schilder, 1935). This is the proposition that every person carries within himself a belief about his personal appearance that results from the interactions between the self and the environment in early childhood. Needless to say, the quality of mothering and the degree of family stability are crucial environmental issues. If the child is reared in a setting of unconditional positive regard, then his reservoir of self-esteem will be ample and the feelings about his appearance will not be disturbing, even in the presence of a serious defect. On the other hand, if the mother, in particular, has problems relating lovingly to the child, then there will appear a vulnerability, a defect in the self-esteem system that may attach itself to a relatively inconsequential assymetry or nasal prominence in an essentially well-formed face. These are the cases that should not be surgically assaulted. These patients may at times be delusionally obsessed with the belief that an actually inconspicuous or even non-existent bodily defect is embarrassingly apparent to others. This condition is called dysmorphophobia (Connolly & Gipson, 1978; Jenike, 1984; Munro & Chmara, 1982). It is also called Monosymptomatic Hypochondriacal Psychosis and it is classified under the heading Atypical Somatoform Disorder (American Psychiatric Association, 1979). This condition is singularly resistant to psychotherapy. However, it does respond to certain psychotropic drugs, namely, tranyl-cypromine, which is available in the United States, and pimozide, which while not available in the United States is obtainable in Europe. These patients are often so eloquent in their plea for surgical help that they may prevail on an even experienced surgeon to operate despite his own better judgment. These patients also make up the so-called recidivist cases, that is, those who seek out surgical revisions of an essentially satisfactory surgical result (Groenman & Sauer, 1983). Here again, the patient's eloquence may prevail and still another ill-advised operation will occur, at times with disastrous medical–legal consequences.

DSM-III

A few words should be said about the current system of disease classification used by the American Psychiatric Association. It is called DSM-III, which stands for Diagnostic and Statistical Manual, Third Edition (American Psychiatric Association, 1979). To the cosmetic surgeon, problems of ter-minology and classifications in psychiatry may seem unimportant. And yet, recent changes have resulted in an important advance which relates funda-mental psychiatric concepts to the rest of medical practice. Although the suggested approach may seem unnecessarily complex at first, the thoughtful reader will be richly rewarded by this ingenious and helpful framework for the consideration of his patients' problems whether they be physical, psycho-logical, or social (Linn, 1983).

DSM-III is a 5-axes approach to patient evaluation (Table 12.1). It is based on the premise that a comprehensive evaluation leading to effective

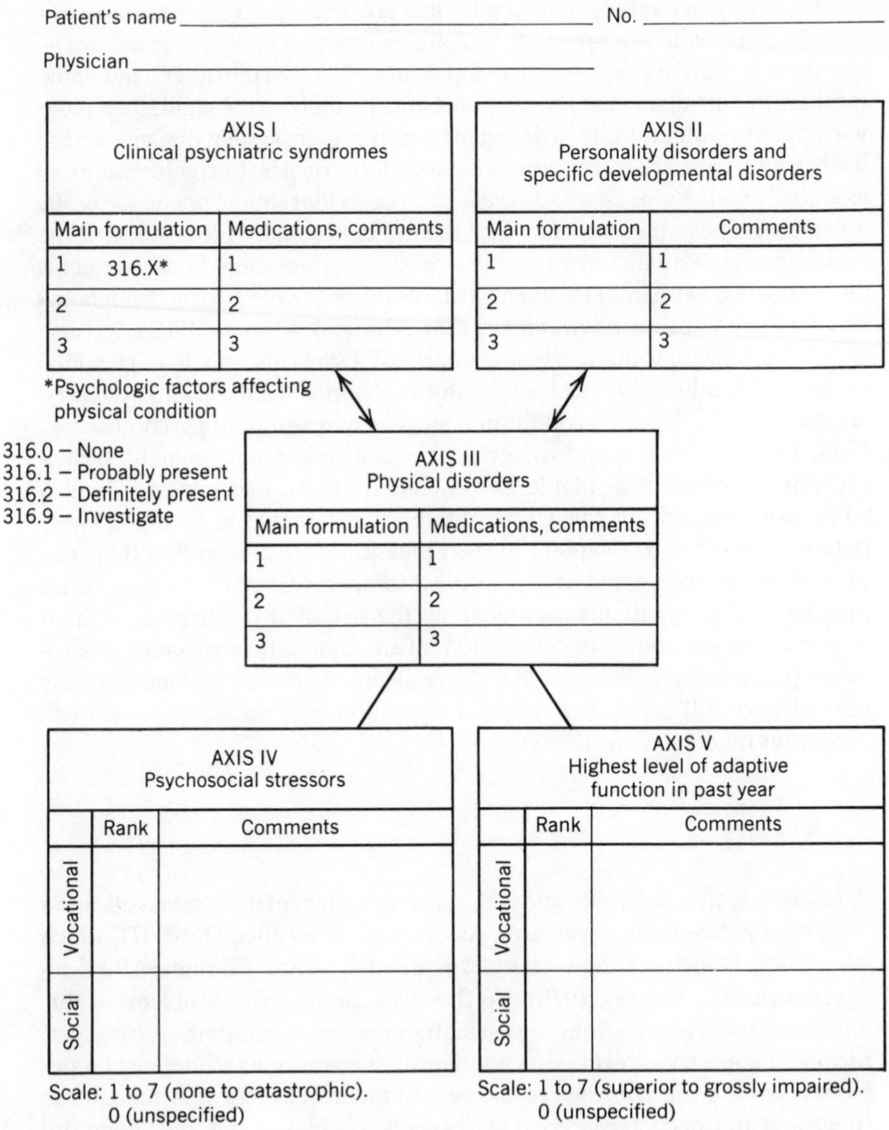

Patient's name _____ No. _____

Physician _____

AXIS I Clinical psychiatric syndromes	
Main formulation	Medications, comments
1 316.X*	1
2	2
3	3

AXIS II Personality disorders and specific developmental disorders	
Main formulation	Comments
1	1
2	2
3	3

*Psychologic factors affecting
 physical condition

316.0 – None
316.1 – Probably present
316.2 – Definitely present
316.9 – Investigate

AXIS III Physical disorders	
Main formulation	Medications, comments
1	1
2	2
3	3

AXIS IV Psychosocial stressors		
	Rank	Comments
Vocational		
Social		

Scale: 1 to 7 (none to catastrophic).
       0 (unspecified)

AXIS V Highest level of adaptive function in past year		
	Rank	Comments
Vocational		
Social		

Scale: 1 to 7 (superior to grossly impaired).
       0 (unspecified)

Figure 12.1. DSM-III "316 Form." *(Source:* Linn, 1983).

treatment involves not only the diagnosis of the patient's physical condition but also consideration of related psychosocial stresses and of the patient's past level of social functioning.

Table 12.1. *Five axes of the DSM-III system of patient evaluation*

Axis I	Clinical syndromes, conditions not attributable to a mental disorder that are a focus of attention or treatment, and additional codes
Axis II	Personality disorders and specific developmental disorders
Axis III	Physical disorders and conditions (as listed in International Classification of Diseases [ICD-9])
Axis IV	Severity of psychosocial stressors
Axis V	Highest level of adaptive function past year

In my opinion, the DSM-III multiaxial system has not only intrinsic interest but profound practical implications for consultants to the cosmetic surgeon. This section briefly discusses the significance of the axes. Axis 3 is introduced first because of its primary importance to the surgeon. It covers all the nonpsychiatric disorders listed in the International Classification of Diagnoses (ICD-9). The cosmetic surgeon would list his diagnosis and planned surgical procedure on this axis. In Figure 12.1, axis 3 is centrally placed to emphasize that these physical issues are of central concern to the nonpsychiatrist physician. However, this figure then tries to force on the nonpsychiatrist the need to consider factors contained on the other four axes. The 316 entry on axis 1 means that there may be some psychological factor affecting the physical condition, and that this possibility should be explored. This is certainly true in every patient who comes for cosmetic surgery and this should be coded (316.2). For example, the previously described condition of dysmorphophobia would also be listed on axis 1 by name and with the official numerical designation 300.70. This entry would alert the surgeon to keep hands off and to refer the patient for psychiatric help, where with appropriate psychotropic medication and supportive psychotherapy the condition might be brought under control.

Reactions of depression would also be listed on axis 1. For many older patients the daily view of one's aging face may intensify and perpetuate a depressed state, secondary, for example, to the loss of a spouse. Patients who have undergone an appropriate period of mourning may decide that the time has come to begin life anew and that help from a cosmetic surgeon may be a good way to start. As a matter of fact, rhinoplasty, rhitidectomy, mentoplasty, and blepharoplasty have all worked well in older patients struggling with reactions of depression.

On the other end of the age scale are adolescent girls who are pushed into rhinoplasty, for example, by overconcerned mothers. Adolescent patients are classically and notoriously in a transitional state, both psychologically and physically. Premature surgery may lead to severe upheavals in this group. In addition, continuing growth of bony nasal structures may lead to undesirable changes in the operated nose.

Whereas axis 1 describes specific clinical syndromes, axis 2 categorizes the ongoing or customary quirks by means of which the patient copes. For example, a patient may display a schizotypal personality disorder, which is characterized by a state of social isolation without friends, with eccentricities of dress, speech, and general behavior that may be so severe at times as to repel the approach of others. In these cases, the personality disorder is calculated to keep a "frightening" world at a safe distance from these mentally disturbed patients. There may be unrealistic family expectations that cosmetic surgery will alter this pattern of social isolation, and when it fails to do so, the family may express dissatisfaction with an essentially successful surgical result.

Case 1

Henry, a 32-year old single, chronically unemployed male patient had a nose with a fleshy tip that was so long that he could pull it down into his mouth and suck on it. As a youngster he was teased as the "elephant boy." He lived at home with his parents. Henry tended to sleep most of the day and would ride the subway trains at night, a pattern he continued despite the fact that he was subjected to muggings on these nocturnal odysseys. By day, he often took solitary bicycle rides. In this case an excellent cosmetic result led as might be expected to no change in his impaired pattern of socializing. He did not get worse but he also did not get better. His parents complained bitterly about this to the surgeon.

Axis 4 asks what social stresses are involved in the patient's request for cosmetic surgery. In other words, it asks the surgeon and the psychiatric consultant "Why now?" This is probably one of the most important questions that the physician can ask (Belfer, Mulliken, & Cochran, 1979).

Case 2

I saw an actor in consultation who had a very successful career playing character roles. A wish to play more romantic roles was the ostensible reason for seeking out cosmetic surgery. However, hidden factors were also involved, complex social and sexual issues that were not considered preoperatively by him or his physicians. When surgery did not help resolve these other issues, the patient lapsed into a severe depression and required psychiatric help. In this case, his decision to seek out surgery occurred when he fell in love with a beautiful leading lady who spurned him and became sexually involved with her romantic leading man. With psychiatric help the patient recovered from his depression and resumed his previous career as a successful character actor. However, his frustrated romantic life was left unchanged.

Case 3

A woman sought out cosmetic surgery in a frantic attempt to save a marriage threatened by her husband's extramarital sexual involvement. A successful surgical result was followed by complicated family upheavals that required long-term psychological and social help for both the patient and her husband.

Case 4

A beautiful married woman decided to correct an essentially imagined nasal assymetry during the second trimester of her pregnancy. She had gained over 40 pounds in the pregnancy. In addition, she and her husband were about to move from a suburban home into a city apartment. During this time she became convinced, falsely, that her husband had entered on a sexual liaison with his former wife. She fought to recapture his love by improving her looks. Despite a minimal and highly skillful surgical intervention, the patient became more deeply convinced than ever that her nose was ugly. This was a classical case of dysmorphophobia that was precipitated by the many changes occurring in her life at one time.

Case 5

A young man about to go to an out-of-town college had a successful rhinoplasty. In college he lapsed into a depression and had to return home. It was clear in retrospect that the young man's fear of separation from his mother precipitated the decision to undergo rhinoplasty. Here again, an unrealistic social expectation was the basis for postoperative dissatisfaction, expectations which could have been identified if the surgeon explored the question "Why now?"

Axis 5 calls for an estimate of the highest level of psychological and social functioning during the preceding year. In the case of the elephant boy, previously referred to, one could have anticipated the limited gains both vocational and social that would have accrued from cosmetic surgery.

It will be noted in Figure 12.1 that axes 4 and 5 are divided into vocational and social components. In the case of the elephant boy, he was unable to function in either category. On the other hand, there are many patients who are outstanding in their vocational careers but totally inept in the conduct of their personal lives, in courtship, marriage, parenting, with friends, and so forth. The actor patient, previously referred to, was outstandingly successful vocationally, but clearly impaired in his social relationships. His postoperative mental breakdown occurred when cosmetic surgery failed to improve his social life. On recovery from his depression he was able to make peace with his limited social success and to derive sufficient self-esteem from his continued successes as an actor. On the other hand, many shy young people may improve enough from cosmetic surgery to venture out more boldly into the world in both the vocational and social spheres. In many of these cases one may speak of the cosmetic improvement as a facilitator of emotional growth. A good job or a fortunate choice of a mate in marriage may lead to further emotional growth and development (the ripple effect). On the other hand, psychotherapy may be needed in some cases to complete the process.

Thus, in psychologically evaluating a candidate for cosmetic surgery, one has to distinguish between vocational goals and social goals and try to ascertain how realistic are the patient's expectations in each of these spheres. Vocational improvement seems to occur more readily than social improvement without the additional help of psychotherapy.

All medical practice should be family centered. Responsible relatives should be involved in these preoperative evaluations. Sometimes the family is unrealistic and sometimes the patient. At times the family joins the patient in unrealistic hopes and expectations that can only be described as a *folie à deux*. In preoperative evaluations it is well to ask the patient if he ever had a "nervous breakdown." The term is vague and is chosen for that very reason. Patients will often give very revealing evidence of emotional instability in responding to that question.

One should also ask the patient if he has ever had psychiatric treatment in the past. If the answer is yes, it is well to call the psychiatrist with the patient's permission. This simple and brief device may be much more fruitful than a consultation with a psychiatrist who is otherwise unfamiliar with the patient.

SUMMARY

The following have been discussed within this chapter:

1. The cosmetic surgeon is participating in an extraordinary psycho-somatic process involving nothing less than a reorganization of the patient's self-concept and his relationship to his entire social network.

2. If a clearly correctable deformity exists, it should be repaired. The odds are clearly good for both the patient and the surgeon. However, beware of the surgical recidivist!

3. In preoperative discussions with the patient he should be told that there may be unforeseen psychological changes. These changes are usually good ones. However, they may at times be anxiety provoking and disappointing. In these instances psychiatric help may be necessary. If there are doubts the patient should be referred to a psychiatrist for preoperative evaluation or treatment. If a case is a questionable one and the patient steadfastly refuses psychiatric consultation, it is advisable to desist from surgery.

4. The most difficult goal in psychiatric treatment is to enhance the patient's capacity to love others. This aspect of life may be enhanced by surgery alone or by fortunate life changes following surgery (the ripple effect). On the other hand, the patient and the surgeon must not be disappointed if postoperative psychological follow up is necessary to fulfill all of the patient's goals.

REFERENCES

American Psychiatric Association (1979). *Diagnostic and Statistical Manual, Third Edition*. DSM–III. Washington, DC: American Psychiatric Association.

Belfer, M. L., Mulliken, J. B., & Cochran, T. C., Jr. (1979). Cosmetic surgery as an antecedent of life change. *American Journal of Psychiatry, 136;* 199–201.

Berscheid, E., & Gangestad, S. (1982). The social psychological implications of facial physical attractiveness. In F. C. MacGregor (Ed.) *Clinics in Plastic Surgery* (pp. 289–296). Philadelphia: Saunders.

Book, H. E. (1971). Sexual implications of the nose. *Comprehensive Psychiatry, 12;* 450–455.

Clark, M., Gosnell, M., Morris, H., Jackson, T. A., Namuth, T., Leerhsen, C., Raine, G., Adler, J., & McCormick, J. (1985, May 27). New bodies for sale. *Newsweek,* pp. 64–71.

Connolly, F. H. & Gipson, M. (1978). Dysmorphophobia—A long-term study. *British Journal of Psychiatry, 132;* 568–570.

DeMoura, L. F. P. (1978). Rhytidectomy (face-lift) in the otolaryngologic practice. *ORL. 86;* 924–929.

Goin, M. K., Burgoyne, R. W., Goin, J. M., & Staples, F. R. (1980). A prospective psychological study of 50 female face-lift patients. *Plastic and Reconstructive Surgery, 65;* 436–442.

Groenman, N. H., & Sauer, H. C. (1983). Personality characteristics of the cosmetic surgical insatiable patient. *Psychotherapy and Psychosomatics, 40;* 241–245.

Jenike, M. A. (1984). A case report of successful treatment of dysmorphophobia with tranylcypromine. *American Journal of Psychiatry, 141;* 1463–1464.

Jensen, S. H. (1978). The psychosocial dimensions of oral and mixillofacial surgery: A critical review of the literature. *Journal of Oral Surgery, 36;* 447–453.

Linn, L. (1983). The DSM-III system as an aid in office practice. *Postgraduate Medicine, 73;* 95–104.

Linn, L., & Goldman, I. B. (1949). Psychiatric observations concerning rhinoplasty. *Psychosomatic Medicine, 11;* 307–314.

MacGregor, F. C. (1982a). Social and psychological studies of plastic surgery: Past, present and future. In F. C. MacGregor (Ed.) *Clinics in Plastic Surgery,* (pp. 283–288). Philadelphia: Saunders.

MacGregor, F. C. (1982b). Surgery: The patient and the surgeon. In F. C. MacGregor (Ed.) *Clinics in Plastic Surgery.* (pp. 387–398). Philadelphia: Saunders.

Munro, A. & Chmara, J. (1982). Monosymptomatic hypochondriacal psychosis: A diagnostic checklist based on 50 cases of the disorder. *Canadian Journal of Psychiatry, 27;* 374–376.

Pertschuk, M. J. & Whitaker, L. A. (1982). Social and psychological effects of craniofacial deformity and surgical reconstruction. In F. C. MacGregor (Ed.) *Clinics in Plastic Surgery.* (pp. 297–306). Philadelphia: Saunders.

Schilder, P. (1935). *The Image and Appearance of the Human Body. (Psyche Monographs No. 4.).* London: Kegan, Paul, French, Trubner and Co.

Schweitzer, I. & Hirschfeld, J. J. (1984). Postrhytidectomy psychosis: A rare complication. *Plastic and Reconstructive Surgery,* (September) 419–422.

— CHAPTER THIRTEEN —

Brief Psychotherapeutic Intervention for the Surgical Patient

RICHARD S. BLACHER, M.D.

It is not surprising that psychological difficulties arise in surgical patients. When one considers the disruption of the patient's normal life as a result of the illness, the hospitalization, the surgery, and the postoperative treatment, it is perhaps more surprising that most patients weather their surgery without difficulty.

When problems do occur, they may create emergency, life-endangering situations. Such events may be overwhelmingly dramatic, as in acute paranoid psychosis postoperatively, or a refusal to consent to a life-saving

Many of the ideas discussed in this chapter were first presented in Blacher, Richard. (1984). The briefest encounter: Psychotherapy for medical and surgical patients. *General Hospital Psychiatry*, 6; 226–232.

procedure. More subtle problems are seen more often, such as quiet depressions where the patient complains of pain, sleeps a great deal, and finds it difficult to move, eat, or cooperate with the medical regimen. When this occurs, the patient is prone to develop deep vein thrombosis, pneumonia, and poor wound healing. Thus, the proper psychological management of these patients may spell the difference between cure and chronic invalidism, or even between life and death.

Unlike the psychiatrist sitting in his office, the physician in charge of these patients does not have the luxury of long-term evaluation and treatment. The nature of the medical emergency demands that treatment be rapid and focused — focused on the problem at hand, while postponing to a later time the leisurely treatment of chronic personality difficulties.

While antipsychotic and antianxiety agents may be useful, and at times even mandatory, much of the treatment to be described in this chapter will emphasize the *psychological* issues, since these are important to (1) understanding what is going on, (2) providing a rational framework for treatment, and (3) ensuring that the underlying conflicts will not serve as a nidus for the further elaboration of neurotic problems lasting well into the future. As with patients seen in traumatic neuroses, such as combat fatigue, the early institution of treatment while there is still a good deal of "psychic fluidity" seems to be effective in preventing the development of chronic conditions.

Two principles should be borne in mind in treating patients in medical and surgical situations. The first is that the current situation may evoke old conflicts and problems concerning the person's relationship to his family, other important objects and to himself. The second principle is that all things have some meaning. If an event causes a reaction seemingly out of proportion to its importance, one must suppose that the *meaning* of the event is of enormous importance to the patient, even though it may seem trivial to the observer.

Case 1

A woman of 53 entered the hospital for relatively minor surgery. Shortly after admission she became markedly agitated for no apparent reason. Her only previous hospitalization had been at the age of 2 when she was stricken with polio and hospitalized at some distance from her family. She rarely saw her parents when hospitalized, and over a period of several years required numerous hospitalizations and operations for the correction of her resultant deformities. For the past 40 years she had functioned well in her everyday life. When it was suggested that her current situation must remind her of her early time in the hospital away from her parents, and all the surgical procedures of those years, her anxiety seemed to fade away and she could recognize that the danger was from the past and not the present.

It is clear that the intrapsychic events which the patient describes are not random. All things have a meaning, and a dynamic understanding becomes important in dealing with the patient's problems.

Some techniques, of course, can bypass understanding and be "imposed" on the patients. But even here, an understanding of what the patient is going through may be extremely useful. Certainly reassurance by the physician can be remarkably effective as a calming agent; exhortation also has its place in mobilizing patients. Hypnosis too is a useful tool on the surgical service, finding its greatest use in allaying pain such as that accompanying major dressing changes when the alternative may be general anesthesia or massive doses of analgesics. At times, hypnosis may also be used to allay anxiety concerning a procedure or even as a form of anesthesia in some surgery— either electively or when another form of anesthesia is considered excessively dangerous.

The use of placebos in the treatment of pain is fraught with some danger on a surgical service. Although placebo use may be effective (Beecher, 1955), its effect on the medical attendants may create all sorts of problems for the patient. A placebo injection will be effective in relieving pain in 35 percent of patients with an injury, such as a leg fracture, yet the staff of most hospitals often do not appreciate this. And if a patient with an obscure pain responds to a placebo, the staff may consider such a patient a faker. In *Pygmalion* George Bernard Shaw (1912) remarked that the difference between a lady and a flower girl is not how she behaves but how she is treated, and this problem of attitude is often reflected in the care of our patients. Instead of sterile water or a sugar pill, a homeopathic dose of an effective agent may be useful as a placebo without endangering the patient's credibility if the medication works.

While a surgical hospitalization may occur in chronically ill psychiatric patients, the underlying psychological problems do not usually create any major problems for the hospital staff. Indeed, patients with major psychotic difficulties may make ideal patients on a general hospital floor unless somebody has learned of their histories, following which the anxiety of the *medical attendants* may mount. If a patient is admitted to the hospital with a history of a psychiatric hospitalization 20 years before, but with normal functioning since, it can be anticipated that there will be an emergency psychiatric consultation requested. Patients with characterological difficulties may create havoc occasionally on certain surgical wards, but most such patients sail through their medical stays with ease.

The patients to be discussed in this chapter are those one might describe as normal–neurotic, whose psychological difficulties stem from the specifics of the surgery as it interplays with their past histories. The treatment will perforce be brief, since so often the psychological difficulty may interfere with the patient's recovery.

Brief psychotherapy was first described in the modern literature by Freud in his *Studies on Hysteria* (Freud, 1895) in the case of Katharina, a young woman he treated with one interview. In recent years, other writers have described brief psychotherapies. Alexander and French (1946), Balint, Ornstein, and Balint (1972), Castelnuovo-Tedesco (1965), De la Torre (1978), Mann (1973), and Sifneos (1972) have all described short-term therapy. But all of these therapies have involved about a dozen interviews spread out over weeks and even months. The techniques to be described will not deal so much with personality issues or with long-standing problems but rather with the disabling and even dangerous reactions that the patient is struggling with currently.

The techniques used will be discussed under the headings of (1) shamanism, (2) cognition, (3) confirmation of reality, (4) speaking the unspeakable, and (5) making the unconscious conscious. Clearly there is an ascending level of sophistication in these treatment headings but such a hierarchy refers to the type of treatment rather than to the psychic level or ego strength of the patients. It is important to bear this in mind, since it is clear that relatively primitive patients might require a sophisticated approach and, at times, high-level functioning patients may respond very well to primitive methods.

SHAMANISM

From the patient's point of view the physician has always stood in the position of shaman and the magical expectation is that the doctor's mere presence will have a curative effect. Despite the accusation that physicians play God they are usually reluctant to take this role, feeling much more comfortable in the position of intellectual explainer. However, there are times when a position of blatant magic-making may be life saving. An occasional example of this is seen in the intensive care unit, when a patient who is suffering a life endangering illness may be unable to sleep. Despite heavy sedation, he lies anxiously awake to the consternation of the doctors and nurses who worry lest this hyperalert state may lead to death. If the surgeon is reluctant to play shaman, it may be left to the psychiatrist to talk to the patient and announce to him "I know that you can't sleep because you are afraid that if you do, you will die. If you do sleep though I can tell you that you will *not* die." The patient will usually respond by asking "How do you know?" and the answer should be "Because we won't *let* you die." On hearing this, the patient usually smiles, relaxes, and falls asleep within a few seconds. Such gross magicianship may be objectionable to many physicians, but it is nevertheless at times lifesaving.

Another shamanistic technique may be called "countermagic." This consists of accepting rather than rejecting the patient's magical expectations and utilizing them in alleviating anxiety (Blacher, 1983). It is important to recognize that most adults in our society are superstitious, having been raised in a culture that encourages such belief, while at the same time intellectually deriding it. Sophisticated patients are more embarrassed about their superstitions, whereas the uneducated openly state their fears. Belief in magic, omens, and luck cuts across all socioeconomic and educational levels, and this regressive focus is common in the crisis of surgery.

Case 2

A 73-year-old retired university educator knew that her anxiety was out of proportion to the risk while awaiting a major operation. Although the procedure was serious it was not considered especially dangerous even for someone her age. She avoided talk of her fears but finally blurted out that she felt she was doomed because of a conversation she had held with her siblings. They had noted that it was remarkable that all five of them had been in excellent health and all were over the age of 65, until the past year when a brother died of a cerebrovascular accident. All of them had agreed that things "would now fall apart," and when questioned about this, she pointed out that her siblings, all highly educated professional people, had agreed that bad things happened in threes, and despite her feeling that she was not superstitious she nevertheless felt that two more would have to die. Since she was facing surgery, it was clear to her that she was next.

At that juncture, it might have been pointed out that such a superstitious concept was nonsense. This of course was a fact with which she would agree. Such a discussion would leave her feeling foolish and embarrassed but still anxious. It would be like attempting to persuade an obsessional that his obsessional symptom makes no sense. This he already knows. The physician therefore decided to play the shaman, and said to her, "I think you are wrong. Since your mother and father died, your brother's death makes the third and therefore closes the circle." To this logically outlandish statement, her response was a broad smile and a nodding of her head "I like your logic" and an obvious lessening of her anxiety. After an uneventful operation she spontaneously remarked to a group of students how the physician's "sensible" approach had made her feel so relaxed before the procedure.

Clearly such shamanistic approaches must be used sparingly. For many physicians such a conscious use of illogical or magical power smacks of charlatanry.

COGNITION

This technique is one used often by all physicians, namely, the giving of correct information. It is a common experience for patients in psychotherapy to *misinterpret* information; the medical patient may just not have the information he needs. The members of the medical staff may take for granted that information they have is common knowledge, yet the patients may not understand what truly occurs. As noted previously, we have seen educated, professional men refusing herniorrhaphy because they did not want their testes removed. They assumed that since the physician had examined them by an exploration of the scrotum, the operation would naturally involve that area. A simple explanation relieves this anxiety and the patient is able to accept surgery. In Chapter Three it was pointed out that patients often have the fantasy that the risk is 50 / 50 in a cardiotomy. The patient may also have the fantasy that the heart is removed from the body during the procedure and that he will be dead while on bypass. A simple explanation and clarification here too is very relieving.

As noted in Chapter One, medical language is very frightening, especially when the words used are those that have meaning in both the vernacular and in technical jargon. Such terms as heart failure and heart block are taken literally by patients, heart block meaning that something blocks blood from going to the heart. A basic scientist in a local medical school, was hospitalized for abdominal pains. She knew nothing about anatomy and became panicky at the physicians' discussion. She surprised a young physician by asking him "Is it true that my ileum is terminal?," and was enormously relieved when the technical terms were translated.

Patients do not know about usual outcomes of procedures, and they often are uncomfortable in asking. They therefore become anxious, for example, when they are not able to speak after a tracheostomy. They imagine that they will never again be able to use their voices, since they may not know that the procedure is reversible. Patients with indwelling urinary catheters who then have difficulty voiding for awhile may imagine that they may never be able to void naturally again. In all of these situations a simple reassurance even when the patient is not able to express his anxiety directly may make life much more tolerable for him.

CONFIRMATION OF REALITY

This technique of therapy involves not only the question of telling the patient the truth but the handling of certain special situations as well. Physicians are constantly in conflict between telling the patient the truth when it involves bad news and trying to hide it when they feel such knowledge will be too anxiety provoking. A popular medical writer of the eighteenth century (Buchan, 1769) pointed out that if one gives the patient a good prognosis and tells the family the ominous truth, the patient has but to take one look at the faces of family members to realize the probable outcome. It is not uncommon to the observer in a recovery room to see that the patient with a negative biopsy has a virtual parade of members of the operating team announcing the results. However, if the biopsy is positive, no one may appear, with the rationalization that the patient is too obtunded to understand what is said. However, in many medical situations the patient fantasizes that the medical condition is far worse than it is in reality. Often, letting the patient know the actual facts can be relieving. For example, during delirium following surgery and resulting from some metabolic disorder, it has been found most useful to confront patients directly with the fact that their minds are not functioning correctly, and to reassure them that when their medical situations are straightened out, they will find their minds working once again. Such patients are often treated as if the loss of brain function has eliminated the psyche, but nothing is further from the truth. Although patients with an organic brain syndrome will not usually admit to their difficulty, their awareness of the dysfunction will create much anxiety and the fear that they may have lost their minds forever. This fear may be seen especially in people with family histories of brain damage.

When Patients Awaken during Surgery

The newer anesthetic agents and muscle paralysants have made it more difficult for the anesthesiologist to know when the patient is actually unconscious, and occasionally we see patients who have awakened sometime during the procedure. Usually we learn about them from the night nurse reporting a patient being confused, anxious, and talking about insanity and knowing what it is like to be dead. These patients reveal, on questioning, that they have repetitive nightmares that are often poorly disguised versions of an operative situation, such as "I'm on the table and people are sticking wires into me." The nightmare may also repetitively express a certain theme, such as "I am always trying to get out of a situation but I just can't move." The predominant affect is one of terror. The patient in such a situation of awakening, usually with an obtunded sensorium, has the feeling that something has gone terribly wrong. Why else would he be awake? At the same time he can not really believe it possible that what he is experiencing is actually occurring. In a sense the patient is in the midst of a nightmare. The repetitiveness of the nightmares indicates that we are dealing with a traumatic situation and treatment consists of telling the patient that during the surgery he had been awake at some time, paralyzed, and unable to move. In our experience the nightmares immediately disappear and the patient is able to resume a normal life, free of symptoms (Blacher, 1975).

Case 3

A 43-year-old accountant underwent mitral valve replacement. Several days after surgery, although he was making very satisfactory physical progress, it was noted that he appeared quite haggard. The night nurse reported that he had been walking around the ward looking somewhat confused. He reported that he had not been able to sleep because his first dream of the night would awaken him in terror. The dreams on succeeding nights were not exactly the same but they had a unifying theme. He would be in some place or situation of grave danger and would seek ways of escaping. However, in all of the dreams escape seemed impossible, and he would awake terrified. It was suggested to him that at some time during the operation he must have been briefly awake and that the feeling of being unable to escape was connected to the sensations he had experienced. His response was to comment that this seemed to make sense. He went back to his room and took a comfortable nap. That night the nightmares did not occur, nor did they recur on any subsequent night.

SPEAKING THE UNSPEAKABLE

This type of therapy involves giving the patient permission to discuss matters that might not ordinarily be found acceptable. The problem for the therapist is being able to decipher what the patient keeps hidden because of the anxiety that his concerns will be considered crazy, critical of the medical profession, or something for which he will be ridiculed. In this category we find those patients, referred to in Chapter Three, whose fantasy is that during the surgery, when their hearts have stopped, they will be dead. It was noted that when one addresses these concerns in a straightforward manner, patients are able to discuss their worries, and seem relieved by the fact that the doctor does not consider them strange for having such thoughts.

Another group of patients in this category is those who are afraid to admit their superstitions concerning the surgical procedure. It is the anticipated danger of the surgery that mobilizes regressive forces and leads to some magical expectation, but patients are worried lest they be laughed at. We see this especially around the anticipation that bad things will happen in threes. Patients who have had two previous surgeries of a similar nature will worry that "Three strikes and you're out" and these patients will be anxious, at times out of proportion to the realistic dangers. We have seen marked anxiety in patients who have had two close loved ones die in the recent past or two members of the immediate family who have died over a period of time. The therapist's mentioning that the patient seems to be worried about this danger of bad things happening in threes, is in itself often reassuring because the patient then feels he will be able to talk about the fear. Other superstitious anxieties include the common fear that the patient is in danger at the time when he is the same age as a parent of the same sex who has died. It is usual that the next birthday is celebrated with the same magical pleasure with which the patients celebrate the fifth anniversary of a cancer surgery A person undergoing a major surgery during this year, fears that the risk is much higher than it actually is, and thus shows an increase in anxiety. Talking about this fear is helpful; at times when the next birthday is near at hand, an elective surgery may even be postponed to allow patients to feel less anxious.

Patients fearing death in surgery often find themselves reluctant to discuss this, lest their worry be construed as a questioning of the surgeon's competence. In dealing with all of these patients it is best to maintain a high level of suspicion and awareness that anxious patients may attempt to hide their worries behind statements of denial or casual utterances.

MAKING THE UNCONSCIOUS CONSCIOUS

For many colleagues this form of therapy is the most challenging and satisfying. More precisely, we should think in terms of making the preconscious as well as the unconscious available. In this treatment, we put into words the conflicts that the patient perforce represses lest their emergence interferes with his staying in the good graces of the surgeon.

Cancellations, Complications, and Other Depressing Events

It is not uncommon on a busy surgical service to have an emergency interfere with the orderly progression of elective procedures. In this case, patients in the least desperate condition may have their operations cancelled — for a day, for several days, or even for a longer period of time. Such patients not uncommonly become depressed. A simple statement that one can understand the frustration of having an operation cancelled after one has prepared oneself psychologically so strenuously, will often suffice to relieve the depression. Even more helpful is the "universalization" of such a reaction. "It seems to me that the natural human reaction to such an event is feeling annoyed and resentful. We all understand that, but also understand that nobody likes to be irritated with the doctors just before they are going to operate on you." Note that the words used are "irritated, annoyed, resentful." Usually it is best not to talk about "anger" or "rage," since these are loaded words for the patient.

Following surgery, one occasionally finds patients with various complications, such as wound infection. These patients also become depressed. They are resentful of the predicament but find such feelings unacceptable because the very people they are angry at are those they count on to cure the condition. In addition, they also like their doctors. Here too we find that the simple statement that one can understand how under these circumstances it would be natural to resent what has happened since an infection is not what one expected or looked for, is usually sufficient to relieve the depression. In this situation also, one gives the patient permission to be angry, to turn the anger outward, knowing that he not in danger from having such feelings toward his medical attendants.

Paranoia

As mentioned in Chapters One and Three, paranoia is not uncommon in many surgical intensive care units. Here the plight of the patient, as a result of the treatment, results in a rage similar to that of the patients just mentioned. However, the nature of his immediate postoperative status results in a greater regression. Thus, instead of turning the anger onto the self as one sees in the depressive reactions, the rage is projected onto the staff. Almost invariably, the paranoia is directed at the nurses rather than at the doctors, since it is *they,* according to his lights, who "torture" him by making him move although it is painful, give numerous injections, and force him to breathe deeply although such breathing is agony. To be angry at the nurses is dangerous because he is at their mercy, and the projection of the rage and resulting paranoia both relieves him of his anger and also explains to him the medical staff's treatment. "I don't want to kill you; you want to kill me. This is why you do these terrible things to me." Often this paranoid reaction is not overt (Blacher, 1972). The best treatment for such paranoia is prevention. If the nurses can give the patient permission to resent the treatment he receives, then there is no need for the patient to project the anger; he can be safe having such a feeling. It should be emphasized that they then *feel* anger but do not express it. It is paranoid patients who in their desperation express their underlying rage in a self-protective way. The nurses give the patients permission by explaining that it's only a natural human reaction to resent something painful even if one knows it is being done for one's own benefit. The liaison psychiatrist may reinforce this idea in talking with the patient. In the cardiac surgery care unit, when such procedures are carried out, it is extremely rare to see a paranoid reaction. (Blacher, 1980).

Postoperative Depression without an Apparent Cause

The emphasis here should be on the word "apparent" since, on careful consideration, there must be a reason for every depressive reaction. All too often, the physician assumes that since the patient has gone through a major procedure, a depressive letdown is a natural consequence. This is not so. A careful investigation will almost invariably reveal the cause of the depression. Not uncommonly after coronary artery bypass surgery we see patients with marked depressions after about the third hospital day. Since a prominent feature of this state is a psychomotor withdrawal and retardation, it presents a danger to the patient's life, as such patients are prone to pneumonia, poor wound healing, venous thrombosis, and pulmonary embolism. Almost invariably these patients give a history of family members who have died of heart disease at an age younger than they are at present. Close questioning will reveal that the patient actually had not expected to live through the operation. The dynamics here, clearly those of survivor guilt (Blacher, 1978; Niederland, 1968), have to do with an unacceptable pleasure in having lived. Our society deals with death in a quantitative way. That is, a certain number of people will live and a certain number of people will die, and if one person dies, it increases the chances of others for survival. The feeling is therefore that one has lived at the expense of the lost objects. In these cases a simple statement can be made that the depression is paradoxical since the patient did not expect to live. One would expect him to be happy that he has lived but we would understand that it must be difficult to celebrate the pleasure of survival when someone one loved has died without a chance such as the patient now has. The usual response to this statement is a nod of the head, and lifting of the depression in the next hour or so.

I would not suggest that the only therapeutic factor here is making an unconscious thought conscious. Rather, other issues may be important. These patients usually do not have a history of depression, and have functioned well previously. In this situation it is as if one loans one's superego to the patient to state to him that the fact of his survival and the deaths of love objects are not connected. In addition, it is suspected that the factor Glover (1955) emphasized in his paper on inexact interpretations probably plays an important role. He suggested that an interpretation that is close to the conflict may be seized upon by the patient in order to avoid a much more upsetting unconscious fantasy. Thus, in this case, the patients do not have to deal with unacceptable death wishes or other issues of conflict with their love objects.

Clearly in this category of patients the role of the history, both personal and family, is important, as it is by this that the therapist can make reasonably informed suppositions about the meaning of the current symptoms. It is not only in coronary bypass surgery that such depressions occur. One sees the same reaction after other major surgical procedures.

Sometimes we see chronic conditions that are also amenable to such treatment.

Case 4

A 52-year-old man became profoundly depressed after a successful gallbladder operation. His medical course had gone smoothly, but he was noted to sleep a great deal and complained of vague generalized pain. When out of bed he would sit motionless in his chair looking sad, and was noted to have no appetite.

He had never had a previous depression. His previous surgeries had included a stormy course following surgery for a benign abdominal condition 10 years before. His history revealed that five years before surgery an older brother had died of a pulmonary embolus several days after gallbladder surgery. The brother was 52 at the time, the same age that the patient was now. It was suggested to the patient that he might have been surprised to have survived the surgery since the brother had died. The patient agreed that this was so. The examiner then said that it must be hard to celebrate having survived an operation that he did not think he would, when someone he loved had died following the same procedure. It was emphasized that his brother's death and *his* living had no real connection although they seemed to him to be associated, and that he had every reason to feel good about having come through his operation so well. Twenty minutes later the patient was observed sitting at the side of his bed eating some sherbet and chatting animatedly with the nurse.

SUMMARY

In none of the interventions described here do we have time to deal with some of the important elements of a good psychotherapeutic situation that we aim for in our offices. First, there is no time to establish the usual therapeutic alliance. Second, transference issues are not dealt with in these therapies although the role of the psychotherapist as an omnipotent figure may be most useful at times and perhaps at all times. A good deal of activity on the part of the therapist is necessary as is good ego strength on the part of the patient. Above all, it would seem that a willingness to be flexible in trying new approaches is useful to the psychotherapist on the surgical floor. A dynamic understanding of the patient and his plight provide this flexibility.

REFERENCES

Alexander, F., & French, T. M. (1946). *Psychoanalytic Therapy: Principles and Application.* New York: Ronald.

Balint, M., Ornstein, P. H., & Balint, E. (1972). *Focal Psychotherapy.* Philadelphia: Lippincott.

Beecher, H. K. (1955). The powerful placebo. *Journal of the American Medical Association, 159;* 1602.

Blacher, R. S. (1972). The hidden psychosis of open heart surgery with a note on the sense of awe. *Journal of the American Medical Association, 222* (3); 305–308.

Blacher, R. S. (1975). On awakening paralyzed during surgery: A syndrome of traumatic neurosis. *Journal of the American Medical Association, 234;* 67–68.

Blacher, R. S. (1978). Paradoxical depression after heart surgery: A form of survivor syndrome. *Psychoanalytical Quarterly, 47;* 267–283.

Blacher, R. S. (1980). "Minor" psychological hazards of critical care. *Critical Care Medicine, 8;* 365–366.

Blacher, R. S. (1983). Clusters of disaster: Superstition and the physician. *General Hospital Psychiatry, 5;* 279–284.

Buchan, J. (1769). *Domestic Medicine.* Edinburgh.

Castelnuovo-Tedesco, P. (1965). *The Twenty Minute Hour.* Boston: Little, Brown.

De la Torre, J. (1978). Brief encounters: General and technical psychoanalytic consideration. *Psychiatry, 41;* 184–193.

Freud, S. (1895). *Studies on Hysteria.* The Standard Edition, Vol. 2, London, Hogarth, 1955.

Glover, E. (1955). *The Technique of Psycho-analysis.* New York: *International Universities Press.*

Mann, J. (1973). *Time-Limited Psychotherapy.* Cambridge, MA: Harvard University Press.

Niederland, W. G. (1968). Clinical observations on the "survivor syndrome." *International Journal of Psychoanalysis, 49;* 313–315.

Shaw, G. B. (1959). Pygmalion. In *Four Plays by George Bernard Shaw* (pp. 213–320) New York: Modern Library. (Original work published 1912.)

Sifneos, P. E. (1972). *Short-term Psychotherapy and Emotional Crisis.* Cambridge, MA: Harvard University Press.

Name Index

221

Subject Index